GUIDE TO MANAGING AN EMERGENCY SERVICE INFECTION CONTROL PROGRAM

2002

UNITED STATES FIRE ADMINISTRATION

As an entity of the Federal Emergency Management Agency, the mission of the U.S. Fire Administration is to reduce life and economic losses due to fire and related emergencies through leadership, advocacy, coordination, and support. We serve the Nation independently, in coordination with other Federal agencies and in partnership with fire protection and emergency service communities. With a commitment to excellence, we provide public education, training, technology, and data initiatives.

PREFACE

In 1992, the United States Fire Administration (USFA) developed the *Guide to Developing an Emergency Service Infection Control Program* in conjunction with the National Fire Academy (NFA) field course, *Infection Control for Emergency Response Personnel: The Supervisor's Role*. These two major Federal initiatives were designed to provide accurate information and guidance to the emergency services regarding communicable disease infection control. Both were developed with the support and assistance of the Centers for Disease Control and Prevention (CDC) and the Occupational Safety and Health Administration (OSHA), to coincide with the promulgation of 29 CFR Part 1910.1030, *Occupational Exposure to Bloodborne Pathogens, Final Rule*.

Since the original publication, many advances have occurred in the field of infection control, and all emergency services should have some form of infection control program. The initial guide focused on the development of an infection control program. The new *Guide to Managing an Emergency Service Infection Control Program* updates relevant information from the original 1992 guide and focuses on the management of an infection control program. The guide is designed to meet or exceed all applicable Federal/national laws, regulations, standards, and guidelines in effect at the time of publication. Many of these are included in their entirety in Appendix B of the guide. The guide also contains Internet Web addresses for accessing those guidelines not included in their entirety.

The principal development team for the guide included: Judy Janing, Ph.D., R.N., EMT-P, Emergency Program Specialist, IOCAD Emergency Services Group, Omaha, NE; Murrey Loflin, M.S., EMT-B, Battalion Chief, Virginia Beach Fire Department, Virginia Beach, VA.; Gordon Sachs, MPA, Director, IOCAD Emergency Services Group; Mike Grill, Captain, Sierra Vista Fire Department, Sierra Vista, AZ; David Barillo, M.D., Associate Professor of Surgery, Medical University of South Carolina, Charleston, SC. Sandy Bodgucki, M.D., Ph.D., Assistant Professor, Yale University School of Medicine, Department of Surgery, Section of Emergency Medicine, New Haven, CT.

Members of the Technical Review Panel for the development of this guide were: Jonathan M. Lieske, M.D., M.P.H., International Association of Fire Fighters (IAFF); Richard Knopf, International Association of Fire Chiefs (IAFC), Health and Safety Committee; Philip Stittleburg, National Volunteer Fire Council; Decker Williams, Phoenix Fire Department; Richard Patrick, VFIS, Inc.; Scott Deitchman, M.D., Centers for Disease Control and Prevention (CDC); Ron Thackery, American Ambulance Association; and Susan McHenry, National Highway Transportation and Safety Administration (NHTSA).

TABLE OF CONTENTS

INTRODUCTION

SCOPE AND PURPOSE

Since infection control requirements vary by agency type, local regulations, department size, etc., emergency response organizations cannot simply adopt a generic infection control program as their program. Therefore, this *Guide* is designed as a resource to help emergency response organizations tailor the requirements identified in regulations and standards to their own unique situations.

The structure of the *Guide* facilitates its use for different purposes. The first section, **Overview of Infection Control** contains two chapters.

- Chapter 1: **Technical Background** summarizes basic terms and concepts, and describes the risks associated with various communicable diseases particularly relevant to emergency services.

- Chapter 2: **Laws and Regulations** summarizes applicable laws, regulations, and standards.

The second section, **Components of an Infection Control Program**, covers the aspects of an infection control program that organizations need to address. These components include risk management, training and education, health maintenance, roles and responsibilities of department personnel, policies and procedures, standard operating procedures, and interactions with other departments.

The third section, **Vehicles, Equipment, and Supply Considerations**, addresses issues related to vehicle design, decontamination of disposable and non-disposable equipment, equipment advances (including needleless systems), and considerations related to clothing/linen and volunteers responding from and returning to home or the primary workplace.

The fourth section, **Facilities Considerations**, discusses infection control in relation to the various functioning areas of emergency services facilities.

The fifth section, **Assessing Effectiveness**, provides a description of the evaluation process. A step-by-step approach for developing performance standards and compliance (evaluation criteria) for measuring effectiveness is described. Other aspects addressed include information management and program revision.

The final section, **Special Situations**, provides a brief overview of infection control practices in the training environment and as they relate to protecting the patient.

In addition, the *Guide* also contains a bibliography of useful reference documents and several appendices:

- **Glossary of Common Terms** used in infection control.

- Text of major **Laws, Standards, and Guidelines** of interest to managers of infection control programs.

- **Sources of Additional Information** for special needs in infection control.

The USFA *Guide* incorporates all requirements specified by applicable regulations and standards at the time of publication. However, users are encouraged to go beyond the information contained in the *Guide* to address specific needs.

Managers also should remember that infection control is a rapidly evolving field. OSHA's *Occupational Exposure to Bloodborne Pathogens*, 29 CFR Part 1910.1030 requires that the department's exposure control plan be reviewed and updated at least annually, and that the consideration and implementation of safer medical devices be documented. It is imperative to review new medical developments, consensus standards, and regulations. This will ensure that mechanisms exist to integrate that new information into a department's existing program. The goal of the infection control program is to provide the best protection available for members.

SECTION 1
OVERVIEW OF INFECTION CONTROL

CHAPTER 1
TECHNICAL BACKGROUND

OVERVIEW

This chapter provides an introduction to the basic principles of infection control in the emergency service environment. Technical terms are defined. The risk of occupational exposure to communicable disease is discussed.

INTRODUCTION TO INFECTION CONTROL

In the mid-1800's in Vienna, Austria, a physician named Ignaz Semmelweis demonstrated the importance of hand washing in decreasing the incidence of infection in women following childbirth. He observed that medical students were conducting cadaver dissections in the morning and then delivering babies in the afternoon without wearing gloves or washing their hands. When the medical students were on vacation, the incidence of infection was reduced. Semmelweis traveled to other European cities to demonstrate that hand washing could reduce deaths related to infection. Even though he had reduced infection from 18 percent to 1 percent in the Vienna hospital, at the time the medical community did not take him seriously.

Although hand washing remains the most fundamental measure for controlling infection, it is still not taken as seriously as it should be. Infection rates in patients, hospital personnel, and emergency responders continue to be a national problem, despite continuing improvements in medical technology.

Infection control procedures have been developed and refined continuously over the years. Unfortunately, research on the incidence of infection, the spread of infection from patient to care provider, and the incidence of infection related to contaminated medical equipment continues to be limited almost exclusively to hospital-based studies. To date, there are few studies related to the incidence of disease in the emergency response environment. As a result, recommended practice and/or procedures for emergency responders are generally modifications of those established for in-hospital personnel.

Without definitive data, it is difficult to demonstrate the need for infection control procedures specifically for emergency services. However, the U.S. Centers for Disease Control and Prevention (CDC) has classified emergency response personnel as being at high risk for exposure. They face the same potential for exposure as hospital personnel.

In many instances, the volatility and unpredictability of the emergency scene increases the level of risk. The *Guidelines for Prevention of Transmission of Human Immunodeficiency Virus and Hepatitis B Virus to Health Care and Public Safety Workers* (MMWR Vol. 38, No. 2-6, 1989) states

> The unpredictable and emergent nature of exposures encountered by emergency and public-safety workers may make differentiation between hazardous body fluids and those which are not hazardous very difficult and often impossible. For example, poor lighting may limit the worker's ability to detect visible blood in vomitus or feces. Therefore, **when emergency medical and public-safety workers encounter body fluids under uncontrolled, emergency circumstances in which differentiation between fluid types is difficult, if not impossible, they should treat all body fluids as potentially hazardous.**

BASIC CONCEPTS

An effective infection control program requires a basic understanding of key infection control concepts.

Disease-Producing Organisms

Viruses and bacteria are the organisms commonly responsible for the spread of disease. Viruses normally reside in a living host and cannot multiply outside of a living cell. However, viruses can spread disease through contact with inanimate surfaces that are contaminated with fluids/blood containing the virus. Bacteria can multiply outside the body, i.e., on surfaces or objects. Therefore, proper cleaning of equipment is critical.

Infectious Versus Communicable Disease

An **infectious** disease results from invasion of a host by disease-producing organisms, such as bacteria, viruses, fungi, or parasites. A **communicable** (contagious) disease is one that can be transmitted from one person to another.

Not all infectious diseases are communicable. For example, there are many cases involving people getting salmonella "food poisoning" from poorly prepared food containing salmonella bacteria. Salmonella is highly infectious, but it is not **contagious**. Chickenpox is an infectious disease that also is communicable. It can be transmitted easily from one person to another by airborne droplets. Infection control for emergency services is primarily, but not solely, concerned with communicable disease.

Modes of Transmission

A communicable disease can be spread directly or indirectly. **Direct transmission** occurs through direct contact with the blood or other body substances of an infected individual. **Indirect transmission** occurs without person-to-person contact; the disease-producing organism passes from the infected individual to an inanimate object. Another person comes in contact with the contaminated object and contracts the disease.

Although a communicable disease may be transmitted by body fluids other than blood (e.g., cytomegalovirus), those of primary concern to emergency responders are those communicable diseases that are bloodborne or airborne. **Bloodborne** diseases are spread by direct contact with the blood or other body substances of an infected person. Bloodborne diseases of most concern to emergency responders include Human Immunodeficiency Virus (HIV), Hepatitis B, and Hepatitis C.

Airborne diseases are spread by droplets of the disease-producing organism being expelled into the air by a productive cough or sneeze or by direct contact with infected bodily secretions. Airborne diseases include tuberculosis, meningitis, mumps, rubella, and chickenpox.

ASSESSING RISK POTENTIAL

Any exposure to a communicable disease carries a certain amount of risk. For bloodborne pathogens, an exposure occurs whenever there is contact with blood or other body fluids through open wounds, mucous membranes, or parenteral (by injection) routes. The degree of risk depends on the degree of exposure. Five factors are critical in assessing potential risk in any exposure situation:

- **Communicability** – Identification of the causative agent is critical. As noted previously, some disease-producing organisms are more readily communicable than others; some are capable of causing more serious effects.

- **Dosage of the Disease-Producing Organism** – Dosage refers to the number of viable (live) organisms received during an exposure. Each illness requires that a certain number of infectious agents be present in order to cause disease. For example, one Hepatitis B virus in 1 milliliter of blood may be all that is needed to spread the infection, while 100,000 HIV viral particles may be needed.

- **Virulence of the Disease-Producing Organism** – Virulence is the disease-evoking power of the organism, in other words, the strength or ability of the organism to infect or overcome bodily defenses.

- **Hardiness of the Organism** – Hardiness is the organism's ability to survive in the environment. This varies from one situation to another. In most cases, the organism must be one that survives outside the body. For example, the hepatitis B virus has been shown to live on a surface for days to weeks and still be infectious.

- **Host Resistance** – Host resistance is the ability of the host to fight infection. Infection occurs as a result of an interruption in the body's normal defense mechanisms, which allows the organism to enter the body. Typically, the healthier you are, the less likely you are to become ill.

BLOODBORNE DISEASES

HIV/AIDS

The number of new HIV cases reported in the United States has decreased slightly over the past decade. CDC reported 47,915 new cases of HIV (17.4 cases/100,000 population) in 1998 and 46,400 new cases (16.7 cases/100,000 population) in 1999. As of the 1999 report, there were 113,000 persons living with HIV and 290,542 persons living with AIDS in the United States. CDC reported twelve potential and no documented cases of HIV in emergency services personnel in 1999. This low number can probably be attributed to the use of personal protective equipment, but it must be remembered that emergency services personnel remain in a high-risk group.

Hepatitis B

Hepatitis B virus (HBV) infection is the major infectious hazard for health-care personnel. The risk of HBV infection after percutaneous exposure varies from 2 percent if the patient is negative for the Hepatitis B early antigen (HBeAg) to 40 percent if HBeAg antigen is present. Overall, the estimated risk of HBV infection after an occupational exposure ranges from 20 to 30 percent.[1] During 1993, an estimated 1,450 workers became infected through exposure to blood and serum-derived body fluids, a 90 percent decrease from the number estimated to have been thus infected during 1985.[2] This decline is partly due to widespread adoption of preventive immunization, increased adherence to universal precautions, and use of personal protective equipment by health-care workers. Hepatitis B immunization is a critical preventative factor of an Emergency Medical Service infection control program.

Hepatitis C

Hepatitis C (HCV) is a leading cause of cirrhosis of the liver, liver cancer, and one of the major causes of the need for liver transplants. CDC estimates that the annual number of newly acquired HCV infections ranged from 180,000 in 1984 to 28,000 in 1995. Of these, an estimated 2-4 percent occurred among health-care personnel who were occupationally exposed to blood. After an unintentional needlestick from an HCV-positive source, the average risk for HCV infection is 1.8 percent. Transmission rarely occurs from mucous membrane exposures to blood, and no transmission has been

---

[1] Swinker, M. (1997). Occupational Infections in Health Care workers: Prevention and intervention. *American Family Physician*, 56 (9), 2291-2303.

[2] U.S. Department of Health and Human Services, Centers for Disease Control. (1997). Immunization of health-care workers: Recommendations of the advisory committee on immunization practices (ACIP) and the hospital infection control practices advisory committee (HICPAC). *Morbidity Mortality Weekly Report*; 46 (RR-18):1-42.

documented from intact or non-intact skin exposures to blood.[3] At least 50-80 percent of persons who contract HCV infection become chronically infected, and half of those chronically infected develop cirrhosis or liver cancer. Up to 10 percent of parenterally transmitted hepatitis may be caused by other bloodborne viral agents not yet characterized.

Hepatitis A

Occupational exposure generally does not increase health-care workers' risk for Hepatitis A virus (HAV) infection.[4] When proper infection control practices are followed, nosocomial HAV transmission is rare. Transmission of HAV from adult patients to health-care workers usually is associated with fecal incontinence in the patients. There is a vaccine for Hepatitis A. Currently it is recommended only for travelers and the military.

Other Hepatitis Viruses

There have been three additional Hepatitis viruses (E, F, and G) identified in addition to Hepatitis A, B, and C. Knowledge regarding these viruses is limited; however it is known that the mode of transmission for E is the fecal-oral route, for G is bloodborne, and F may be bloodborne.

Risk of Infection

Risk of infection from bloodborne diseases varies according to the type of exposure. The following list was published by the CDC to help evaluate risk levels. Risk decreases from top to bottom.

---

[3] U.S. Department of Health and Human Services, Centers for Disease Control. (2000). Hepatitis C virus infection among firefighters, emergency medical technicians, and paramedics - Selected Locations, United States, 1991--2000. *Morbidity Mortality Weekly Report*; 49 (29); 660-665.

[4] U.S. Department of Health and Human Services, Centers for Disease Control. (1997). Immunization of health-care workers: Recommendations of the advisory committee on immunization practices (ACIP) and the hospital infection control practices advisory committee (HICPAC). *Morbidity Mortality Weekly Report*; 46 (RR-18):1-42.

- Contaminated needle stick injury (large-bore, hollow needle carries more risk than small bore solid needle).

- Cuts with sharp objects covered with blood/body fluid.

- Blood/Body fluid contact with an open area of the skin.

- Blood/Body fluid contact to the mucous membrane surface of the eyes, nose, or mouth.

- Blood/Body fluid contact to intact skin.

Although incidence of the major bloodborne diseases have decreased over the past several years, emergency service personnel remain at risk for contracting these diseases. If these declines are to be sustained, emergency service personnel must continue to adhere to protection strategies.

AIRBORNE DISEASES

Tuberculosis (pulmonary)

The airborne disease of greatest concern to emergency services providers is tuberculosis (TB). Nationally, the number of reported cases of TB increased by 14 percent from 1985 to 1993. Consequently, concern about this disease increased, and more attention was focused on control measures. At the same time drug-resistant tuberculosis also increased, creating a serious concern. From 1982 to 1986, only 0.5 percent of new cases were resistant to both isoniazid and rifampin. By 1991, this proportion had increased to about 3.1 percent. Among recurrent cases, 3.0 percent were resistant to both drugs during the 1982 to 1986 period, but in 1991 this proportion had more than doubled, to 6.9 percent.

The reported cases of TB began a decline in the years following this increase. There were 26,673 cases (10.5/100,000 population) in 1992. This decreased to 17,531 cases (6.4/100,000 population) in 1999. Of the cases reported in 1999, 2.5 percent occurred in health-care workers. Statistics specific to emergency services are not available, since CDC does not break out emergency services workers as a separate category in their TB surveillance program.

Drug-resistant cases also have decreased. In 1999, 12.2 percent of new cases and 8.4 percent of recurrent cases were resistant to isoniazid alone and 3.8 percent of new cases and 1.1 percent of recurrent cases were resistant to both isoniazid and rifampin.

It is well known that the organism that causes TB dies when exposed to light and air, however there are factors that can affect the potential for infection from TB as well as other airborne diseases. These factors are duration of exposure and ventilation. Some diseases require prolonged exposure in order to contract the disease. Therefore shorter transport times can reduce risk potential. Risk potential also can be reduced by maximum ventilation. Ventilation systems for vehicles are addressed in depth in Section 3 of this *Guide*. On older vehicles without modern ventilation systems, personnel should open windows whenever possible.

INFECTION CONTROL TECHNIQUES

Hand washing is the most effective overall infection control measure, yet it is frequently ignored. Hands should be washed whenever gloves are removed, after all patient contacts, and after disinfecting equipment, as well as before eating and after using the bathroom. Hands should be well lathered with regular soap and scrubbed for at least 15 seconds before rinsing and drying. The towel should be used to turn off the faucet.

Universal precautions is an infection control strategy developed by the CDC for **hospital workers**. Specific precautionary procedures are recommended for reducing potential exposure to bloodborne pathogens. Universal precautions are based on the concept that blood and **certain** body fluids (any body fluids containing visible blood, semen, vaginal secretions, tissues, cerebrospinal fluid (CSF), synovial fluid, pleural fluid, peritoneal fluid, pericardial fluid, and amniotic fluid) of all patients should be considered potentially infectious for HIV, HBV, HCV, and other bloodborne pathogens.

In 1996, CDC published **standard precautions**. Standard precautions synthesize the major features of body substance isolation and universal precautions and apply to isolation precautions in **the hospital setting**.

Body substance isolation (BSI) goes beyond universal precautions and considers **all** body substances potentially infectious. Thus, in addition to those listed under universal precautions, feces, nasal secretions, sputum, sweat, tears, urine, and vomitus also are considered potentially infectious. Such an approach obviously is safer in the emergency response environment, where medical histories are often incomplete or not known at all and differentiation between body fluids may be impossible. In effect, each emergency incident has exposure potential.

BSI is generally accomplished through the barrier technique, using personal protective equipment (gloves, masks, protective eyewear, gowns, and resuscitation devices) to prevent personal contact with blood or other potentially infectious materials. Other infection control techniques include proactive preventive measures such as health maintenance, immunization programs, decontamination procedures, proper waste handling and disposal practices, and both initial and ongoing training.

SUMMARY

The intent of this chapter was to provide a brief overview of communicable disease and infection control principles, as background information for the rest of the *Guide*. Table 1-1-1, on the following pages, summarizes the most common communicable diseases encountered by emergency services personnel.

It must be emphasized that a crucial component of an effective infection control program is learning as much as possible about various types of communicable disease and updating the infection control program as new knowledge becomes available. Organizations should capitalize on all available expertise by enlisting the help of local health and medical practitioners and/or infection control experts. Additional sources of information are provided in the References and Bibliography, and in Appendix C.

Table 1-1-1
DISEASE INFORMATION FOR EMERGENCY RESPONSE PERSONNEL

Disease/Infection	Mode of Transmission	Vaccine Available	Signs/Symptoms	Post-Exposure Treatment
AIDS/HIV (Human Immunodeficiency Virus)	Needlestick, blood splash into mucous membranes (e.g., eyes, mouth), or blood contact with open wound	NO	Fever, cough, night sweats, weight loss,	Antiretroviral Regimen (see complete guidelines in Appendix B)
Chickenpox (Varicella)	Respiratory secretions and contact with moist vesicles	YES	Fever, rash, cutaneous vesicles (blisters)	Vaccine
Diarrhea: **Campylobactor Cryptosporidium Giardia Salmonella Shigella Viral Yersinia**	Fecal/Oral	NO	Loose, watery stools	None
German Measles (Rubella)	Respiratory droplets and contact with respiratory secretions	YES	Fever, rash	Vaccine in 72 hours, immune globulin
Hepatitis A (HAV)	Fecal/Oral	YES	Fever, loss of appetite, jaundice, fatigue	Immune globulin, vaccine
Hepatitis B (HBV)	Needlestick, blood splash into mucous membranes (e.g., eye or mouth), or blood contact with open wound. Possible exposure during mouth-to-mouth resuscitation	YES	Fever, fatigue, loss of appetite, nausea, headache, jaundice	Booster and/or immune globulin

DISEASE INFORMATION FOR EMERGENCY RESPONSE PERSONNEL (cont'd)

Disease/Infection	Mode of Transmission	Vaccine Available	Signs/Symptoms	Post-Exposure Treatment
Hepatitis C (HCV)	Same as Hepatitis B	NO	Same as Hepatitis B	None
Hepatitis D (HDV)	Same as Hepatitis B dependent on HBV (past or present) to cause infection	NO	Same as Hepatitis B	None
Hepatitis E,F, & G	Several viruses with different modes of transmission	NO	Fever, headache, fatigue, jaundice	None
Herpes Simplex (Cold Sores)	Contact of mucous membrane with moist lesions. Fingers are at particular risk for becoming infected.	NO	Skin lesions located around the mouth	
Herpes Zoster (Shingles) localized disseminated (See Varicella)	Contact with moist lesions	Varicella vaccine may be effective even if person has already had varicella	Skin lesions, regional associated pain	
Influenza	Airborne	YES (changes yearly based on strains expected to cause infection)	Fever, fatigue, loss of appetite, nausea, headache	Antivirals (amantadine, rimantadine, zanamivir, and oseltamivir)

DISEASE INFORMATION FOR EMERGENCY RESPONSE PERSONNE L (cont'd)

Disease/Infection	Mode of Transmission	Vaccine Available	Signs/Symptoms	Post-Exposure Treatment
Lice: Head, Body, Pubic	Close head to head contact. Both body and pubic lice require intimate contact (usually sexual) or sharing of intimate clothing.	NO	Severe itching and scratching, often with secondary infection. Scalp and hairy portions of body may be affected. Eggs of head lice (nits) attach to hairs as small round, gray lumps.	Wash clothes, personal articles in hot water.

Gamma benzene hexachloride shampoo (Kwell, Rid, etc.) if crawling lice or nits are noted close to the scalp. |
| **Measles** | Respiratory droplets and contact with nasal or throat secretions | YES | Fever, rash, cough | See German Measles |
| **Meningitis:**

Meningoccocal | Respiratory secretions contact | YES | Fever, severe headache, stiff neck, sore throat, may have distinctive rash | Rifampin, Cephlosporin |
Haemophilus influenza (usually seen in very young children)	Respiratory secretions contact	YES	(Same)	
Viral	Fecal/Oral	NO	(Same)	
Mononucleosis	Contact with respiratory secretions or saliva, such as with mouth-to-mouth resuscitation	NO	Fever, sore throat, fatigue, swollen lymph nodes/spleen	

DISEASE INFORMATION FOR EMERGENCY RESPONSE PERSONNEL (cont'd)

Disease/Infection	Mode of Transmission	Vaccine Available	Signs/Symptoms	Post-Exposure Treatment
Mumps (Parotitis)	Respiratory droplets and contact with saliva	YES	Fever, swollen salivary (parotid) glands	See German Measles
Salmonellosis	Foodborne	NO	Sudden onset of fever, abdominal pain, diarrhea, nausea, and frequent vomiting	
Scabies	Close body contact	NO	Itching, tiny linear burrows or "tracks," vesicles - particularly around fingers, wrists, elbows, and skin folds	
Syphilis	Primarily sexual contact; rarely through blood transfusion	NO	Genital and cutaneous lesions, nerve degeneration (late)	
Tuberculosis, pulmonary	Airborne	NO	Fever, night sweats, weight loss, cough	Isoniazid Rifampin, pyrazinamide
Whooping Cough (Pertussis)	Airborne, direct contact with oral secretions	YES	Violent cough at night, whooping sound when cough subsides	

Note: Post-exposure protocols change frequently based on new information. The Centers for Disease Control and Prevention (CDC) and the *Morbidity Mortality Weekly Report* should be checked regularly for the most up-to-date information.

CHAPTER 2

LAWS, REGULATIONS, AND REGULATIONS

OVERVIEW

A formal infection control program has two basic goals: (1) to provide all members with the best possible protection from communicable disease; and (2) to protect patients from potential infection. A resultant third goal is to protect the department or jurisdiction from potential liability. A properly designed infection control program will help reduce the risk of members contracting a communicable disease, manage civil liability, lower health insurance costs, minimize "sick time," and ensure compliance with all applicable statutes. Knowledge of applicable laws, regulations, and standards is a prerequisite to meeting these goals. This chapter summarizes current national laws, regulations, and standards that relate to emergency service infection control.

LAWS, REGULATIONS, AND STANDARDS

Many Federal and national organizations play a critical role in establishing requirements and recommendations for infection control in the work environment. These organizations include:

- Public Law (U.S. Congress)
- The Occupational Safety and Heath Administration (OSHA), U.S. Department of Labor
- The National Fire Protection Association (NFPA)
- The U.S. Department of Health and Human Services, Centers for Disease Control and Prevention (CDC).

Ensuring compliance with the standards described in this *Guide* is crucial in managing an effective infection control program. However, additional research will be needed to identify State and/or local regulations that also apply.

While State/local regulations vary from jurisdiction to jurisdiction, some of the more common ones include

- **Duty-to-act laws** that require emergency response personnel to provide a "reasonable level of care" to all patients.
- **Patient abandonment laws** that specify that patient care may be relinquished only to someone having an equal or higher level of medical expertise.

- **Biohazard waste laws** that govern the storage, handling, and disposal of medical waste.

PUBLIC LAW

Ryan White Comprehensive AIDS Resources Emergency Act of 1990 (PL 101-381)

This act delineates specific notification requirements that allow emergency response personnel to find out if they have been exposed to an "infectious disease" while providing patient care. Diseases covered include Hepatitis B, tuberculosis, meningococcal (bacterial) meningitis, and HIV.

Each employer of emergency response personnel is required to name a "designated officer" to coordinate communication between the treating facility (hospital) and the emergency response organization. Notification of exposure may be "routine" or "by request."

Routine notification - Notification must be provided by the treating facility to the designated officer when it is determined that a patient transported by emergency response personnel has an airborne communicable disease. This includes patients that expire in transit, or shortly after. Notification must be made no later than 48 hours after the diagnosis is made. Routine notification only pertains to transportation crews. It does not cover responders who provide on-scene care but not transportation.

Notification by request - Any member who "attended, treated, assisted, or transported" a victim of an emergency where exposure to infectious disease may have occurred can request notification. The request is made through the designated officer, who reviews the case and notifies the treating facility. The treating facility reviews the case and notifies the designated officer that: a) an exposure took place; b) an exposure did not take place; or c) insufficient information exists to determine exposure risk. In disputed cases, or cases of insufficient information, the designated officer may use the services of the local public health officer in resolution. This Act does not authorize mandatory patient testing for infectious diseases.

Americans with Disabilities Act (ADA) (PL 101-336)

This Act provides a national mandate for the elimination of discrimination against individuals with disabilities. The ADA prohibits discrimination against disabled individuals in the areas of hiring, firing, promotion, benefits, and management of staff. The ADA obligates employers to make **reasonable accommodation** to the disabilities of otherwise qualified people, in order to guarantee equal employment opportunities.

"Contagious diseases," such as tuberculosis and HIV infection, are considered disabilities under the ADA. People with contagious (communicable) diseases are protected against discrimination, as long as they can perform the essential functions of a job and do not pose a threat to the health and safety of others in the workplace. Cases must be considered individually; one individual who has a communicable disease and poses a serious health threat does not justify excluding all persons with actual or perceived communicable diseases.

Fear expressed by other employees of being infected by an "otherwise qualified" employee with a communicable disease must be supported by objective evidence of risk. If a person poses a significant risk of transmission of infection that cannot be eliminated by reasonable accommodation, the person may be found to constitute a direct threat to the health or safety of others.

The ADA poses a substantial potential liability to any employer who fails to heed the requirements of the Act. Lawsuits and/or fines may be a result of discriminatory acts in hiring, firing, promotion, benefits, and/or management of staff. Compliance may be costly, and must be considered in budgetary planning. This includes training of employees, supervisors, and managers if necessary.

Health Care Worker Needlestick Safety and Prevention Act (PL 106-430)

Passed unanimously by Congress, the Needlestick Safety and Prevention Act became effective in November 2000. This Act directed OSHA to make specific revisions to the *Occupational Exposure to Bloodborne Pathogens* (29 CFR Part 1910.1030) within 6 months. These revisions went into effect January 18, 2001 with the release of *Occupational Exposure to Bloodborne Pathogens; Needlesticks and Other Sharps*

Injuries; Final Rule (29 CFR Part 1910.1030). The text of the law can be found in Appendix B1.

OSHA REGULATIONS

The Occupational Safety and Health Administration (OSHA), U.S. Department of Labor, is the branch of the Federal government responsible for safety in the workplace. OHSA publishes Federal regulations that establish minimum standards for workplace safety and health. Each State, territory, or possession has the option of adopting OSHA regulations as published, or enacting "State" OSHA plans that are at least as stringent as the Federal standards. Table 1-2-1 lists the States that have their own OSHA plans.

Table 1-2-1

STATES/TERRITORIES WITH OSHA PLANS

Alaska	Michigan	South Carolina
Arizona	Minnesota	Tennessee
California	Nevada	Utah
Connecticut	New Jersey	Vermont
Hawaii	New Mexico	Virginia
Indiana	New York	Virgin Islands
Iowa	North Carolina	Washington
Kentucky	Oregon	Wyoming
Maryland	Puerto Rico	

Applicability

Emergency service personnel are not always covered by OSHA regulations. Determining whether or not a particular agency is required to comply with OSHA regulations requires research. However, the following general guidelines apply.

Federal OSHA regulations generally apply only to Federal, military, and private employers. Thus, in States that have simply adopted the Federal OSHA regulations, most emergency service personnel (whether paid or volunteer) are not covered.

If a State opts to develop its own OSHA plan, all paid State and local government employees (including emergency response personnel) **must** be covered. (In some States, only State and local employees are covered.) However, each specific State decides whether or not to include volunteer emergency response personnel. At present, 24 States, the Virgin Islands, and Puerto Rico have "State" OSHA plans. OSHA maintains a list of States with their own plans and contact information on their Web site at http://www.osha.gov/as/opa/worker/.

Emergency response personnel involved in hazardous material response in States and territories having a State OSHA plan are covered under OSHA 29 CFR Part 1910.120. For workers not covered by a State OSHA plan, the Environmental Protection Agency (EPA) issued a regulation (40 CFR Part 311) in 1989. This regulation is functionally similar to OSHA's Hazardous Waste Operations and Emergency Response (HAZWOPER) regulation, specifically citing that the requirements in the OSHA 29 CFR Part 1910.120 will be applicable in all States, regardless of OSHA status.

Communicable disease risks and hazards are the same in each State, regardless of local compliance requirements. Thus, adherence to OSHA regulations is recommended for **all** emergency service agencies.

Occupational Exposure to Bloodborne Pathogens (29 CFR Part 1910.1030)

This regulation establishes standards for workplace protection from bloodborne diseases. The primary diseases of concern are Hepatitis B (HBV), Hepatitis C (HCV), and Human Immunodeficiency Virus (HIV). The primary methods of protection are training, engineering and work practice controls, immunization against HBV, and the use of universal precautions. Recognizing that the tasks performed by emergency responders often are undertaken during uncontrolled situations, the regulation states that **all body fluids are considered infectious when differentiation between fluid types is difficult.**

Each employer must establish an "exposure control plan." The plan must

- Identify and categorize all job classifications and tasks that reasonably can be anticipated to have a potential for exposure to blood or body fluids.
- Delineate the implementation plan and schedule for the infection control program.

- Identify the procedures for evaluating/investigating exposure incidents.

This regulation prohibits eating, drinking, smoking, applying cosmetics, or handling contact lenses in work areas where there is potential for occupational exposure to bloodborne pathogens. Hands must be washed as soon as feasible after removal of gloves or other personal protective equipment. If hand-washing facilities are not available (e.g., at the scene), alternative hand-washing provisions must be provided by the employer.

Personal protective equipment (PPE) is covered in detail. Employers are required to supply, repair, and replace PPE including gloves, gowns, face shields or masks and eye protection, and resuscitation equipment. Exemptions to the use of PPE are allowed where "its use would have prevented the delivery of health-care of public safety services or would have posed an increased hazard to the safety of the worker or co-workers." These exemptions are meant to apply to unexpected, "rare and extraordinary circumstances." The decision not to use PPE rests with the employee, and not the employer.

A general framework for post-exposure care that follows Public Health Service guidelines is presented, including the need for medical recordkeeping. Each employee must receive a copy of the regulation and, to assure understanding, must receive training in communicable disease/infection control. Written training records must be maintained, including attendance. Training must be provided annually in each of the following subjects:

- Epidemiology, modes of transmission, and symptoms of bloodborne diseases.
- The employer's exposure control plan.
- Recognition of tasks that may result in exposure to bloodborne diseases.
- Use and limitations of practices that will reduce or prevent exposures.
- Proper selections, use, location, removal, handling, decontamination, and disposal of PPE.
- Information on Hepatitis B vaccine.
- Emergency procedures, including post-exposure requirements.
- Recognition of standard biohazard markings, color-coding, and labeling.

Subpart Z of *Occupational Exposure to Bloodborne Pathogens; Final Rule.* (OSHA 29 CFR Part 1910.1030) are included in Appendix B2. The entire regulation is available on the Web at http://www.osha-slc.gov/OshStd_data/1910_1030.html.

Occupational Exposure to Bloodborne Pathogens; Needlesticks and Other Sharps Injuries; Final Rule (29 CFR Part 1910.1030, January 18, 2001)

This regulation updates the original *Occupational Exposure to Bloodborne Pathogens* (29 CFR Part 1910.1030) to include the requirements of the Health Care Worker Needlestick Safety and Prevention Act (PL 106-430). This adds new requirements for exposure control programs and requires the use of a sharps/needlestick injury log. The revision clearly specifies engineering controls necessary for minimization of employee exposure. It clarifies the need to involve employees in identifying and choosing the devices and includes provisions designed to maintain the privacy of employees who have experienced needlesticks. The text of this regulation can be found in Appendix B3 of this manual and also is available on the Web at http://www.osha-slc.gov/needlesticks/index.html.

Access to Employee Exposure and Medical Records (29 CFR Part 1910.20)

This section provides for employee access to their own medical and exposure records and regulates the storage of such records. Employers must make medical and relevant exposure records available within fifteen days of any formal request. A physician representing the employer may recommend that the records be released as a summary rather than the complete chart, or that the records be released only to a physician. This section also allows OSHA access to medical and exposure records.

Employee medical/exposure records must be maintained for the duration of employment plus thirty years. Instruction on transfer of records is provided for businesses that close before the thirty-year limit is reached.

NATIONAL FIRE PROTECTION ASOCIATION (NFPA)

Standards and codes published by the NFPA represent the consensus opinions of a committee of experts representing different interests relating to the subject matter involved. NFPA standards are not mandatory until official adoption by the authority having jurisdiction. Nor does NFPA enforce or monitor compliance. However, since NFPA standards reflect the national "industry standard" or "standard of care", a department not meeting these standards could face possible liability in the event of litigation.

NFPA 1500 (1997 Edition)

NFPA 1500, *Standard on Fire Department Occupational Safety and Health Program*, is an umbrella document intended to establish a framework for a comprehensive safety and health program. It requires an official written department occupational safety and health policy, and the appointment of an occupational safety and health officer, an occupational safety and health committee, and a fire department physician. Health maintenance issues addressed include pre-entry health examinations and periodic health reassessment as specified in NFPA 1582, *Standard on Medical Requirements for Fire Fighters and Information for Fire Department Physicians*, and after "debilitating illnesses or injuries."

Infection control recommendations include active attempts to identify and limit member exposure to contagious diseases and making available "inoculations, vaccinations, and other treatment." It requires departments to operate an infection control program as specified in NFPA 1581, *Standard on Fire Department Infection Control Program*, and to maintain a confidential health database that documents occupational injuries, illnesses, and exposures to hazardous materials, toxic products, or contagious diseases.

Preventive health measures recommended include a member assistance and wellness program and a critical incident stress program. Recordkeeping requirements and confidentiality safeguards for member assistance programs are listed.

NFPA 1521 (1997 Edition)

NFPA 1521, *Standard on Fire Department Safety Officer*, differentiates between the roles of Incident Safety Officer (ISO) and Health and Safety Officer (HSO). The Health and Safety Officer must "have and maintain a knowledge of the current health and physical fitness factors" that affect the work environment. The Health and Safety Officer has the authority to "cause immediate correction of situations that create an imminent hazard to members." The Incident Safety Officer must "have and maintain a knowledge of safety and health hazards involved in emergency operations" and has the authority to "alter, suspend, or terminate" activities at an emergency incident that are judged to be "unsafe or to involve an imminent hazard."

The standard also requires the establishment of a department database to maintain records of all "accidents, occupational deaths, injuries, illnesses, and exposures." The Health and Safety Officer is responsible for management and analysis of this information.

NFPA 1581 (2000 Edition)

NFPA 1581, *Standard on Fire Department Infection Control Program*, establishes minimum requirements for an infection control program in emergency service organizations. Specific areas addressed include

- Program components, including the designation of an Infection Control Officer.
- Station facilities and apparatus requirements.
- Personal Protective Equipment.
- Cleaning, disinfection, and disposal procedures.
- Post-exposure procedures.
- Immunization requirements.

Immunization requirements vary somewhat from CDC recommendations. CDC currently recommends immunizations for Hepatitis B, measles, mumps, rubella, influenza, and chickenpox. NFPA recommends immunization for Hepatitis B and influenza, and "where specific or local conditions dictate": Hepatitis A, measles, mumps, rubella, tetanus and diptheria (Td) booster every 10 years, and meningococcal disease.

NFPA 1582 (2000 Edition)

NFPA 1582, *Standard on Medical Requirements for Fire Fighters and Information for Fire Department Physicians*, addresses the medical requirements necessary for persons who perform firefighting tasks. Two categories of medical conditions are identified. Category A identifies the medical conditions that "would not allow a person to perform firefighting operations." Category B identifies medical conditions that must be evaluated "on a case-by-case basis" to determine if the condition would prevent a person from performing firefighting operations.

The standard specifically requires "a tuberculosis monitoring program that will test members at least annually and as indicated by CDC guidelines." Medical evaluations, medical examinations, recordkeeping, and confidentiality also are addressed.

CENTERS FOR DISEASE CONTROL AND PREVENTION

The Centers for Disease Control and Prevention (CDC) publishes the *Morbidity Mortality Weekly Report* (MMWR), a weekly update of information on communicable diseases. The infection control officer should review periodically MMWR for new information. A subscription is expensive; however, the contents are available for both the latest and past issues of MMWR online at http://www2.cdc.gov/mmwr/mmwr_wk.html. Liaison with a local infection control practitioner is another possible source of current information. The most current issues dealing with worker protection from HIV, HBV, HCV, tuberculosis, and immunization recommendations are summarized on the following pages. All of the MMWR publications discussed in this *Guide* can be viewed and downloaded in Adobe format in their entirety by accessing the "Search" at http://www2.cdc.gov/mmwr/mmwr_wk.html and typing in the Volume, Number, and Date.

Recommendations for Prevention of HIV Transmission in Health-Care Settings (MMWR Vol. 36, No. 2, August 21, 1987)

This document established the concept of "universal precautions." Under universal precautions, the blood and certain body fluids of **all** patients are considered potentially infectious. Although saliva still has not been implicated as a mode of transmission for HIV, the use of mouthpieces or resuscitation bags to minimize the need for mouth-to-mouth resuscitation was recommended.

Additional information is available from CDC regarding respiratory protection against tuberculosis. *CDC Recommendations from Respiratory Protection* updates the 1994 recommendations to account for subsequent national Institute for Occupational

Safety and Health (NIOSH) respiratory classifications and contains the recommendation for respirators meeting Class N95 or better. This document is available at http://www.cdc.gov/niosh/tb.html. NIOSH also has produced several reference documents on this subject, including *Protect Yourself Against Tuberculosis* (http://www.cdc.gov/niosh/tb.html) and *Respiratory Protection Program In Health Care Facilities – Administrator's Guide* (http://www.cdc.gov/niosh/99-143.html).

Universal Precautions for Prevention of Transmission of Human Immunodeficiency Virus, Hepatitis B Virus, and Other Bloodborne Pathogens in Health Care Settings (MMWR Vol. 37, No. 24, June 24, 1988)

This document extended universal precautions to include body tissues and cerebrospinal, synovial, pleural, pericardial, and amniotic fluids. Universal precautions are not required for feces, nasal secretions, sputum, saliva, urine, tears, or vomitus, unless they contain visible blood.

Blood was cited as the most important source of HIV/HBV infection in occupational settings. Semen and vaginal secretions also can transmit HIV/HBV as sexual diseases.

Guidelines for Prevention of Transmission of Human Immunodeficiency Virus and Hepatitis B Virus to Health Care and Public Safety Workers (MMWR Vol. 38, No. 2-6, 1989)

This document was published in response to the Health Omnibus Programs Extension Act of 1988 (PL 100-607). Universal precautions were expanded to the extent that "when emergency medical and public-safety workers encounter body fluids under uncontrolled, emergency circumstances in which differentiation between fluid types is difficult, if not impossible, they should treat all body fluids as potentially hazardous." This document is often considered the "Bible" of emergency service infection control. However, much of the information contained in these guidelines was taken from other MMWR's.

Recommendations for Preventing Transmission of Human Immunodeficiency Virus and Hepatitis B Virus to Patients During Exposure-Prone Invasive Procedures (MMWR Vol. 40, No. RR-08, July 12, 1991)

This document addresses the status of health-care workers who have HIV or HBV. Although directed at hospital personnel, this document identifies exposure-prone procedures as those that include digital palpation of a needle tip in a body cavity or the simultaneous presence of the health-care worker's fingers and a needle or other sharp instrument or object in a poorly visualized or highly confined anatomic site.

The document also outlines the scope of practice for infected health-care workers as follows. Health-care workers who are infected with HIV or HBV (and are positive for the HbeAg antigen) should not perform exposure-prone procedures unless they have sought counsel from an expert review panel and been advised under what circumstances, if any, they may continue to perform these procedures. Such circumstances would include notifying prospective patients of the health-care worker's seropositivity before they undergo exposure-prone invasive procedures.

Health-care workers whose practices are modified because of their HIV or HBV infection status should, whenever possible, be provided opportunities to continue appropriate patient-care activities. Career counseling and job retraining should be encouraged to promote the continued use of the worker's talents, knowledge, and skills. Health-care workers whose practices are modified because of HBV infection should be reevaluated periodically to determine whether their seropositive status changes due to resolution of infection or as a result of treatment

Guidelines for Preventing the Transmission of Mycobacterium Tuberculosis in Health-Care Facilities, 1994 (MMWR Vol. 43, No. RR-13, October 28, 1994)

This document updates the 1990 guidelines and focuses on the importance of a) the hierarchy of control measures, including administrative and engineering controls and personal respiratory protection; b) the use of risk assessments for developing a written tuberculosis (TB) control plan; c) early identification and management of persons who have TB; d) TB screening programs for health-care workers; e) health-care worker training and education; and f) the evaluation of TB infection control programs. The following criteria are identified for respiratory protective devices:

- "The ability to filter particles 1 um in size in the unloaded state with a filter efficiency of greater than or equal to 95percent (i.e., filter leakage of less than or equal to 5 percent), given flow rates of up to 50 L per minute.
- The ability to be qualitatively or quantitatively fit tested in a reliable way to obtain a face-seal leakage of less than or equal to 10 percent.
- The ability to fit the different facial sizes and characteristics of health care workers, which can usually be met by making the respirators available in at least three sizes.
- The ability to be checked for face piece fit, in accordance with standards established by the Occupational Safety and Health Administration (OSHA) and good industrial hygiene practice, ... each time they put on their respirators."

Two recommendations specific to emergency medical services are

- "When EMS personnel or others must transport patients who have confirmed or suspected active TB, a surgical mask should be placed, if possible, over the patient's mouth and nose. Because administrative and engineering controls during emergency transport situations cannot be ensured, EMS personnel should wear respiratory protection when transporting such patients. If feasible, the windows of the vehicle should be kept open. The heating and air-conditioning system should be set on a nonrecirculating cycle.
- EMS personnel should be included in a comprehensive PPD screening program and should receive a baseline PPD test and follow-up testing as indicated by the risk assessment. They should also be included in the follow-up of contacts of a patient with infectious TB."

Immunization of Health-Care Workers: Recommendations of the Advisory Committee on Immunization Practices (ACIP) and the Hospital Infection Control Practices Advisory Committee (HICPAC) (MMWR Vol. 46, No. RR-18, December 26, 1997)

This report discusses all the immunizations recommended for health-care workers and provides the regime for those immunizations. ACIP strongly recommends that all health-care workers be vaccinated against (or have documented immunity to) Hepatitis B, influenza, measles, mumps, rubella, and varicella.

The report identifies Hepatitis B virus (HBV) infection as the major infectious hazard for health-care personnel. Prevaccination serologic screening for prior infection is not indicated. Postvaccination testing for antibody to Hepatitis B surface antigen (anti-HB's) response is indicated for health-care workers who have blood or patient contact and are at ongoing risk for injuries with sharp instruments or needlesticks. Studies among adults have demonstrated that, despite declining serum levels of antibody, vaccine-induced immunity continues to prevent clinical disease or detectable viremic HBV infection. Therefore, booster doses are not considered necessary. This is a change from the 1990 recommendations. Table 1-2-2 summarizes these recommendations.

Table 1-2-2
Immunization of Health-Care Workers: Recommendations of the Advisory Committee on Immunization Practices (ACIP) and the Hospital Infection Control Practices Advisory Committee (HICPAC)

Disease	Immunization	Notes
Hepatitis B	Series of three doses	Mandated by OSHA that it is offered to employees at employer's expense.
Influenza	Yearly in the fall	Each year influenza vaccine recommendations are reviewed and amended to reflect updated information concerning influenza activity in the United States for the preceding season. These recommendations are published annually in the MMWR, usually during May or June.
Measles, Mumps, Rubella	Series of two doses	MMR is the vaccine of choice.
Varicella	Series of two doses	Recommended for all health-care workers
Tetanus, Diptheria	Primary vaccination of previously unvaccinated adults consists of three doses of adult tetanus-diphtheria toxoid.	Booster is recommended every 10 years. When wound is incurred, booster should be administered if last booster was more than 5 years prior.

ACIP does not recommend routine immunization of health-care workers against tuberculosis, Hepatitis A, pertussis, meningococcal disease, typhoid fever, or vaccinia. However, immunoprophylaxis for these diseases may be indicated in certain circumstances.

Catch-Up Vaccination Programs

Managers of health-care facilities should consider implementing catch-up vaccination programs for those already employed, in addition to policies to ensure those newly hired receive necessary vaccinations. This strategy will help prevent outbreaks of vaccine-preventable diseases. Because education enhances the success of many immunization programs, reference materials should be available to assist in answering questions regarding the diseases, vaccines, and toxoids, and the program or policy being implemented.

Updated U.S. Public Health Service Guidelines for the Management of Occupational Exposures to HBV, HCV, and HIV and Recommendations for Postexposure Prophylaxis (MMWR, Vol. 50, No. RR-11, June 29, 2001)

This report updates and consolidates all previous U.S. Public Health Service recommendations for the management of health-care workers who have occupational exposure to blood or other body fluids that might contain Hepatitis B (HBV), Hepatitis C (HCV), or HIV.

Recommendations for HBV postexposure management include initiation of Hepatitis B vaccine series to susceptible unvaccinated persons and Hepatitis B immune globulin and/or Hepatitis B vaccine series after evaluation of the Hepatitis B surface antigen status.

Immune globulin or antiviral drugs are not recommended for HCV. However, the HCV status of the source person and the exposed person should be determined. If the source person is positive, follow-up testing should be conducted to determine if an infection develops.

Recommendations for HIV include a basic 4-week course of two drugs (zidovudine [ZDV] and lamivudine [3TC]; 3TC and stavudine [d4T]; or didanosine [ddI] and d4T). For exposures that pose an increased risk of transmission, an expanded regimen includes the addition of a third drug. The complete text of this guideline is included in Appendix B4.

SUMMARY

The department infection control program is designed to protect both the health of the members and the department against related liability. For these reasons, it is important to review and remain current on Federal, State, and local statutes affecting infection control/environmental issues.

Infection control is a rapidly expanding field. As new knowledge is gained, the laws, standards, and regulations based on this knowledge will change. The department Infection Control Officer needs to stay up-to-date on both medical and legal changes. The department plan must be reviewed and revised to incorporate these changes at appropriate intervals.

SECTION 2

COMPONENTS OF AN INFECTION CONTROL PROGRAM

INTRODUCTION

Developing, implementing, and managing an effective and efficient infection control program is a process that involves several key components. After it is developed, changes continually take place that require the program be updated and revised to provide the best protection possible for members.

RISK MANAGEMENT

Risk management is comprised of many elements including liability, insurance, safety, health, security, financial impact, and several others. The risks encountered by emergency services personnel are many, such as traffic, response hazards, blood and body fluids, and violence. To control these risks effectively, a fire or EMS department must use a risk management program. **The primary focus of the internal (organizational) risk management plan is firefighter safety and health.**

Occupational exposure to blood, body fluids, or communicable or infectious disease is a very real hazard for department members on a daily basis. A written infection control policy or program is one essential component that must be incorporated into the risk management plan. Regardless of the type of service delivery (first responder, Basic Life Support (BLS), or Advanced Life Support (ALS)), departments need to have an infection control program and a risk management plan.

The safety and health component of risk management was incorporated into NFPA 1500, *Standard on Fire Department Occupational Safety and Health*, during the 1992 revision process. Simply stated, the requirements of the risk management program are

- The fire department shall adopt an official written risk management plan which addresses organizational policies and procedures.

- The risk management plan shall be developed to address the following areas: administration, facilities, training, vehicle operations, protective clothing and equipment, operations at emergency incidents, operations at non-emergency incidents, and other related activities.

- The risk management plan shall include the following components:

- risk identification
- risk evaluation
- risk control techniques
- risk monitoring

There is an additional step that can be added or incorporated into this process, which is typically inserted between the risk identification and risk control techniques. This step is called **prioritization of risks**.

RISK MANAGEMENT MODEL

There is no single method or solution for managing risk effectively. Determining how to manage risk is a decision each department should make based on the risk management model. In order for the risk management plan to be effective, the following components must be included

Risk Identification:　　　Actual or potential hazards for all job functions.

Compile a list of all emergency and non-emergency operations provided by the department. There are many sources to assist with this identification process. The first, and possibly the most effective, is the department's loss prevention data.

Risk Evaluation:　　　The potential of occurrence of a given hazard and the severity of its consequences.

Once the risks are identified, they can be evaluated from the standpoint of both frequency and severity. Frequency addresses the likelihood of occurrence. Typically, if a particular type of incident, such as back injuries have occurred repeatedly, they will continue to occur until effective control measures are implemented.

Severity addresses the degree of seriousness of the incident. This can be measured in a variety of ways such as time away from work, cost of damage, cost of and time for repair or replacement, disruption of service, or legal costs. Using the information gathered in the identification step, the risks then can be classified based on severity.

Prioritizing Risk: The degree of a hazard based upon the frequency and severity of occurrence.

Taken in combination, the results of the frequency and severity determinations will help to establish priorities for determining action. Any risk that has a high probability of occurrence combined with serious consequences, deserves immediate action, and would be considered a high priority item. On the other end of the scale, non-serious incidents with a low likelihood of occurrence are a lower priority, and can be placed near the bottom of the "action required" list.

Risk Control Measures: Solutions for elimination or reduction of real or potential hazards by implementing an effective control measure.

There are several approaches for controlling risk, including risk avoidance, implementation of control measures, and risk transfer.

In any situation, the best choice is **risk avoidance.** Simply put, this means avoid the activity that creates the risk. Frequently in an emergency services organization this is not a practical choice. Lifting a patient onto a stretcher presents a serious back injury risk, but you cannot avoid this risk and still provide effective service!

An example of where avoidance has been very practical is the widespread use of sharps containers. The risks associated with recapping needles are well documented, so recapping is no longer an accepted practice. This risky behavior can be avoided through the proper use of a sharps container.

The most common method used for the management of risk is the adoption of effective **control measures.** While control measures will not eliminate the risk, they can reduce the likelihood of occurrence or mitigate the severity. Safety programs, ongoing training and education programs, and well-defined standard operating procedures (SOP's) are all effective control measures.

Some typical measures instituted for infection control include appropriate use of personal protective equipment (PPE) (gloves, masks, goggles, etc.) during patient contact, training and education, and competent SOP's. The combined use of these control measures results in an effective program that reduces the risk of exposure to infectious disease. **Risk transfer** can be accomplished in two primary ways - physically transferring the risk to somebody else, or through the purchase of insurance. For a fire or EMS organization, the transfer of risk may be difficult, if not impossible. However, examples of risk transfer would be 1) scheduling a routine transfer patient in protective isolation in a newer vehicle with circulating air rather than an older vehicle, and 2) contracting out the laundering of contaminated linen/clothing to a commercial laundry. The risks associated with example two have been transferred to a private contractor.

The purchase of insurance transfers financial risk only. It does nothing to affect the likelihood of occurrence. Buying fire insurance on the station, while highly recommended to protect the assets of the department, does nothing to prevent the station from burning down. Therefore, insurance is no substitute for effective control measures.

Risk Monitoring: Evaluation of effectiveness of risk control
                          measures.

The last step in the process is risk management monitoring. Once control measures have been implemented, they need to be evaluated to measure their effectiveness. Any problems that occur in the process have to be revised or modified. This final step ensures that the system is dynamic, and will facilitate periodic reviews of the entire program.

The intent of the risk management plan is to develop a strategy for reducing the inherent risks associated with fire department operations. Regardless of the size or type of fire department, every organization should operate within the parameters of a risk management plan. This is a dynamic and aggressive process that must be monitored and revised annually by the health and safety officer.

The risk to members providing care to a patient with a communicable disease poses a real hazard and should be properly addressed through a written infection control program. The infection control program should include, at a minimum, the following issues:

- Training and education
- PPE
- Health maintenance
- Immunizations

- Exposure management
- Fire department facilities
- Fire department vehicles
- Cleaning, disinfecting, and disposal

Infection control is a preventive means of controlling risks associated with patient care. By incorporating infection control into the risk management process, frequency and severity of risks associated with communicable diseases are adequately controlled. The health and safety officer, designated infection control officer, incident safety officer, and the department's Occupational Safety and Health Committee should ensure that evaluations and revisions to the risk management plan occur at least annually.

Safety is a major component of risk management. Most of the emphasis placed on risk management from a fire service perspective is from a safety approach. The safety component affects other risk management components in areas such as liability and finance. An aggressive, proactive occupational safety and health program will reduce accidents, injuries, occupational illnesses, and health exposures. This, in turn, reduces the department's liability claims and payments and also provides a positive effect on the financial well being of the organization. Many fire departments are self-insured, which means that the entity, jurisdiction, or the fire department generates funding for various types of insurance such as workers' compensation, vehicle and general liability.

TRAINING AND EDUCATION

Training and education is a vital component to ensure a successful program, and is a crucial element of the risk management process. The department shall conduct initial and annual training and education programs for all members in accordance with Federal or State regulations. Members will receive bloodborne pathogen training at the time of initial assignment of job functions (recruit training or company in-service) whenever exposure potential exists. Additional training shall be provided whenever there are changes in work assignments, job functions, or new protective clothing and equipment is placed in service. Training will include an opportunity for members to have their questions answered by the instructor.

Topics for the infection control training program include

- Epidemiology
- Proper use of PPE
- SOP's for safe work practices relating to infection control
- Proper methods of disposal of contaminated medical waste
- Cleaning and decontamination
- Reporting process of exposures
- Exposure management.
- Medical followup care and treatment.

All training and education programs for infection control will be properly documented in writing. The training report needs to include

- Dates of training session
- Contents and/or summary of the training session
- Names and qualifications of instructor(s)
- Names and job titles of members attending.

MEMBERS

Each member of the fire department has the right to be protected by an effective occupational safety and health program and shall participate and comply with the requirements of the occupational safety and health program. Each member can also participate or be represented in the research, development, implementation, evaluation, and enforcement of this program.

The infection control program has the goal of identifying the risks of exposures to members and the means to prevent those exposures. All members have the individual responsibility for their own health, safety, and welfare. Each member is responsible for complying with all departmental SOP's, including occupational safety and health. Each member must ensure his or her own safety and health against occupational exposures by:

- Participating in available health maintenance programs (annual medical examinations, immunizations, medical screenings, etc.)
- Practicing good personal hygiene
- Reporting any personal medical conditions which could require work

restrictions

- Following infection control procedures at emergency incidents or while conducting patient care at any time

- Properly using all infection control protective clothing and equipment

- Reporting and documenting all exposures

- Complying with medical followup treatment

- Assuring proper decontamination of equipment after each incident

- Proper storage/disposal of contaminated waste

- Attending annual retraining of all members as required by *Occupational Exposure to Bloodborne Pathogens* (29 CFR Part 1910.1030).

HEALTH MAINTENANCE

All members of fire departments and emergency medical services organizations must participate in a health maintenance process. The health maintenance program is a significant part of the infection control process. The health maintenance process as it relates to infection control includes

- Access to an appropriate immunization program which includes immunization against influenza and Hepatitis B;

- Members shall be offered immunizations for the following:
  - Hepatitis A
  - Measles, Mumps, and Rubella
  - Tetanus/Diptheria
  - Meningococcal disease
  - Other diseases as required by specific incidents or local conditions

- Access to tuberculosis screening on an annual basis.

- Health maintenance program which complies with NFPA 1582, *Standard on Medical Requirements for Fire Fighters and Information for Fire Department Physicians.*

- The development of a confidential health database is established and maintained for each member in accordance with NFPA 1582, *Standard on Medical Requirements for Fire Fighters and Information for Fire Department*

Physicians and 29 CFR Part 1910.20, *Access to Employee Exposure and Medical Records.*

- In the event of an exposure, the member shall receive a confidential medical evaluation, post-exposure prophylaxis, counseling, and evaluation.

- Return-to-work policy.

ROLES AND RESPONSIBILITIES

Many different individuals within a department or organization have a valuable role to ensure that the infection control program is developed, implemented, and properly and effectively managed. Each individual must understand his/her role and responsibility in this process for the safety, health, and welfare of the members. Role definition must spell out specific areas of responsibility and accountability throughout the organization. Specific role definitions will vary in each department, depending on organizational structure, available resources, and program requirements. The most vital issue is assigning and managing the necessary components of the infection control program.

Chief of the Department

Although the chief of the department may have little direct involvement in daily operations, he/she has the ultimate responsibility for the health and welfare of department members. The chief of the department is responsible for ensuring that an infection control program has been developed and implemented, adequate funding is available for the training, resources, procurement of equipment, supplies, and health maintenance requirements. The chief must ensure that adequate staffing is available to accomplish program goals and objectives and must define authority and responsibility for each position identified in the infection control program. In addition, he/she has the ultimate responsibility of holding each member accountable for assigned functions.

Safety Officer

The Safety Officer is defined by two distinct functions - Health and Safety Officer (HSO) and Incident Safety Officer (ISO). Each of these job functions has a defined responsibility relating to infection control. In larger departments, the HSO serves as the manager of the department's occupational safety and health program, while the ISO is assigned to particular shifts or at emergency incidents to manage the operational issues relating to firefighter health and safety. In smaller departments, the Safety Officer may have both titles, as well as the additional title of infection control officer.

Health and Safety Officer

The HSO has the responsibility of ensuring that the department has an effective occupational safety and health program. As the manager of this program, the HSO is responsible for ensuring that the fire department's infection control program meets the requirements of 29 CFR Part 1910.1030, *Occupational Exposure to Bloodborne Pathogens*, 29 CFS Part 1910 *Occupational Exposure to Bloodborne Pathogens; Needlesticks and Other Sharps Injuries; Final Rule, Guidelines for the Management of Occupational Exposures to HBV, HCV and HIV and Recommendations for Postexposure Prophylaxis* (MMWR, May 15, 2001), and NFPA 1581, *Standard on Fire Department Infection Control Program*.

If the department does not have an infection control officer, the HSO fills this void. If the department does have an infection control officer, the HSO maintains a liaison with this individual to assist in achieving the objectives of the infection control program as required by NFPA 1581, *Standard on Fire Department Infection Control Program*.

Incident Safety Officer

As an operational function, the ISO monitors for compliance at an emergency incident. The ISO can monitor emergency operations relating to infection control. The ISO must ensure compliance with NFPA 1581, *Standard on Fire Department Infection Control Program* during EMS operations. Any problems that are encountered relating to infection control can be channeled through the HSO for changes in appropriate areas such as SOP's, training and education, and PPE.

Infection Control Officer

The Ryan White Comprehensive AIDS Resource Emergency Act of 1990 requires each department to name a designated infection control officer. One of the primary responsibilities of the infection control officer is to serve as a liaison between the department and the treating facility in a potential or actual exposure.

The infection control officer should be a member of the department's occupational safety and health committee. The infection control officer works closely with the HSO and the ISO to ensure compliance with program goals. The infection control officer is responsible for ensuring the availability of PPE, monitoring compliance, and quality assurance throughout the department, as well as maintaining required documentation and recordkeeping.

Chief of Training

The chief of training is responsible for ensuring that all members have met their initial and annual training requirements as required by 29 CFR Part 1910.1030, *Occupational Exposure to Bloodborne Pathogens*, 29 CFS Part 1910 *Occupational Exposure to Bloodborne Pathogens; Needlesticks and Other Sharps Injuries; Final Rule*, and NFPA 1581, *Standard on Fire Department Infection Control Program*. Each member must demonstrate the necessary knowledge, skills, and abilities required to perform his/her assigned tasks safely and to meet the mandated laws and standards.

The chief of training must work with the HSO and the infection control officer to ensure a competent training program. Program managers must be provided with an overview of the entire program. Officers must receive training in SOP's, compliance, monitoring, recordkeeping requirements, and proper use of protective clothing and equipment.

Occupational Safety and Health Committee

Each department should establish an occupational safety and health committee. This committee provides an avenue for department members to voice their concerns regarding safety and health issues, provide guidance to the HSO, participate in research and development projects, and suggest development of policies and procedures related to occupational safety and health. The primary purpose of the committee is to study, review, and make recommendations pertaining to occupational health and safety within a department. Objectives of this committee should include

- Review department health and safety issues related to SOP's
- Research and make recommendations concerning all fire department related equipment
- Review causes of accidents and injuries within the department and develop means of reducing these incidents
- Develop and implement an infection control program which meets the applicable laws, codes, and standards
- Effect a reciprocal flow of information to all department members as it pertains to health and safety.

The occupational safety and health committee will be involved with policy development, research of proper PPE, make recommendations for facility safety issues, and participate in training programs. The participation and involvement by members of this committee brings expertise that improves the safety and health within the department.

Field Supervisors/Company Officers/Battalion Chiefs

All supervisors in the department are responsible for supporting, promoting, and ensuring that each member comply with the infection control program. Leading by example is a key component of the leadership and management required for a compliant infection control program. First-line supervisors play a critical role in this process by serving as a positive role model. The supervisor's attitude and behavior relating to infection control have a profound influence on actions or inactions of subordinates.

Supervisors must ensure that all components of the infection control plan are properly followed, particularly:

- Health maintenance (assuring members are fit for duty)
- Notification and documentation of exposures
- Storage, maintenance, and availability of all necessary supplies, protective clothing, and equipment

- Training

- Decontamination and waste disposal

- Proper use of protective clothing and equipment.

Supervisors also have the responsibility for managing an incident scene, including ensuring effective customer service when dealing with citizens, maintaining patient confidentiality, and being sensitive to the needs of the patient.

Fire Department Physician

The fire department physician is responsible for developing, implementing, and managing a health maintenance program that is compliant with the requirements of NFPA 1582, *Standard on Medical Requirements for Fire Fighters and Information for Fire Department Physicians*. This process involves a comprehensive health maintenance program for all members, which includes 1) pre-entry and ongoing health assessments, 2) immunizations, 3) postexposure procedures, 4) recordkeeping, 5) medical treatment and followup care, and 6) member assistance program.

The size and needs of the organization will dictate whether the fire department needs a full-time physician. Fire departments of all sizes and types, including those that do not provide EMS, should have a working relationship with at least one designated physician who can serve as the primary medical contact with other physicians and specialists. Alternately, a department can designate several physicians, use the services of a group practice, or have multiple providers -- whichever best meets the needs of the organization and its members. The most important aspect is to have a physician who is aware of the medical needs of the department members and who is available on an immediate basis.

The fire department physician is responsible for guiding, directing, and advising members regarding their health and fitness to perform assigned duties and responsibilities. He/She oversees the health components of the department's occupational safety and health program and serves as a resource for the infection control officer, particularly in assessing potential exposure incidents.

Another key requirement is to be available for consultation and counseling following members' exposures. The physician should provide objective information regarding risk of disease based on specific type of exposure, potential risk to members' families, recommended followup treatment, possible long-term effects of the disease, and prophylactic therapy. Maintaining confidentiality is an important responsibility of the fire department physician.

The fire department physician should have specific expertise and experience relating to the needs of firefighters and emergency medical personnel and a thorough knowledge of the physical demands involved in emergency operations. If possible, he/she should be a specialist in the field of occupational medicine.

Local Medical Facility

The local medical facilities (hospitals) must have procedures in place which provide adequate feedback to the department regarding exposures to a communicable disease. The medical facility's infection control officer must work jointly with the department's infection control officer so feedback in either direction will ensure the health and welfare of the members. The process must enable members to report a potential or actual exposure to the department's infection control officer. This individual forwards the information to the medical facility's infection control officer for proper action. If the medical facility determines a patient has a communicable disease (e.g. tuberculosis), this information must be passed onto the responders who treated and transported the patient. Immediate notification must be made by the medical facility's infection control officer to the department's infection control officer. Exposures occur at various times, and the notification process must be functional 24 hours a day/7 days a week in order to meet the medical requirements specified for testing, prophalyxsis, and reporting.

Municipal/County Risk Manager

Those fire and EMS departments that are self-insured must provide the funding for workers' compensation, medical care and treatment, medical followup, and other components of the infection control process funded by the government entity. A funding process must be established to ensure the program is financially capable of maintaining this program. If fire and EMS departments carry private insurance, these costs are covered by the insurance policy. Prevention is a key to the success of the infection control program. A risk manager prefers to fund a preventive program rather than the financial impact of long-term or chronic health problems or conditions.

POLICIES AND PROCEDURES

NFPA 1581, *Standard on Fire Department Infection Control Program*, requires that a fire department develop and implement a written infection control plan and *Occupational Exposure to Bloodborne Pathogens* (29 CFR Part 1910.1030) requires the department to have a written exposure control plan. For members to practice effective control procedures and practices, the department must have a written infection policy statement and procedures. Simply stated, the goal of the infection control plan is to identify and limit the exposure of members to communicable or infectious disease during the course of their assigned duties and while in fire department facilities.

Policy Statement

The policy statement discusses purpose, scope, and content and sends a safety and health message regarding the severity of the issue to all members. Figure 2-1 is an example of an infection control policy statement.

Figure 2-1

Virginia Beach Fire Department
Virginia Beach, VA
Infection Control Program
Policy Statement

Purpose: To provide control measures to prevent an exposure to a communicable disease during the delivery of patient care.

Scope: To provide specific procedures that comply with the requirements of 29 CFR Part 1910.1030, *Exposure to Bloodborne Pathogens* and NFPA 1581, *Standard on Fire Department Infection Control Program.*

These procedures define the minimum requirements for an infection control program.

In order to have a successful program, this plan utilizes the primary components of 29 CFR Part 1910.1030 and NFPA 1581. These components include engineering and work practices controls, personal protective clothing and equipment, training, medical surveillance, vaccinations, hazard communication, and risk management.

It is the policy of the department to:

- The goal of this policy is to provide all members with the best available protection from an occupational exposure to a communicable disease.

- To provide fire, rescue, and emergency medical services to the public without regard to known or suspected diagnoses of communicable disease in any patient.

- To provide all members with the necessary immunizations and personal protective equipment (PPE) needed for protection from communicable diseases.

- To regard all patient contacts as potentially infectious.

- To regard all medical information as strictly confidential. No member health information will be released without signed consent of the member.

- Training will be conducted annually regarding infection control procedures and practices.

- Each member is responsible for his or her safety and health and the department will provide as safe a workplace as possible.

EXPOSURE CONTROL PLAN

An exposure control plan is designed to minimize and prevent the exposure of department members to infectious diseases transmitted through human blood, body fluids, and other potentially infectious materials. The *Occupational Exposure to Bloodborne Pathogens*, 29 CFR Part 1910.1030 requires an exposure control plan. The exposure control plan encompasses all members who must comply with the requirements of an infection control program. The exposure control plan compliments the specific procedures of individual departments. All members with a reasonable potential for exposure to blood, body fluids, and other potentially infectious materials as part of their assigned job tasks are included in the exposure control plan.

The basic components of the exposure control plan include

- Exposure Determination
- Methods of Compliance
- Hepatitis B Vaccination Policy
- Procedures for Evaluation and Followup
- Exposure Incidents
- Member Training
- Recordkeeping Procedures

The exposure control plan mandates that the employer identify those tasks and procedures with the potential for an occupational exposure. The employer also must identify the positions in the department with duties and responsibilities that may result in an occupational exposure. Lastly, the exposure control plan requires the employer to identify the members who will receive training, protective clothing and equipment, vaccination, and other benefits of the OSHA *Occupational Exposure to Bloodborne Pathogens* regulation.

The exposure control plan will be designed to include an implementation schedule and methods of compliance with the OSHA *Occupational Exposure to Bloodborne Pathogens* regulation. Once the written program is in place, the employer is charged with providing copies to all members. Initial and annual update training must be conducted. Training also must be conducted as needed to educate members about new or modified changes to procedures which affect infection control practices or changes in member duties and responsibilities.

STANDARD OPERATING PROCEDURES

A SOP is defined as an organizational directive that establishes a course of action. A fire department uses a SOP to provide the necessary control measures to prevent an occupational exposure to a communicable disease.

Topics that should be covered in an infection control SOP are training and education, health maintenance, PPE, respiratory protection, eye protection, operational procedures, handling sharps, skin washing, facility disinfecting and cleaning areas, disinfecting and cleaning of equipment, disinfecting and cleaning vehicles, biohazard waste, exposure incidents and medical follow-up, and the infection control officer. The U.S. Fire Administration's *Developing Effective Standard Operating Procedures for Fire and EMS Departments* (1999) is an additional resource for information regarding SOP's. It can be downloaded from http://www.usfa.fema.gov/usfapubs/.

INTERACTION WITH OTHER DEPARTMENTS

With the implementation of an infection control program, the fire department should have interaction with other city or county public safety agencies. These agencies face similar problems and issues relating to compliance with infection control standards and regulations. Combining resources and efforts will improve this process for all members involved. As a city or county entity develops a comprehensive infection control program, an exposure control plan can incorporate all applicable departments.

Law Enforcement

Law enforcement agencies face a variety of issues relating to infection control. Police, sheriffs, and other law enforcement departments must consider the same infection control factors as a fire and EMS department. Compliance may be more difficult due to work schedules, station and precinct locations, proper cleaning, disinfecting and disposal facilities, and type of services provided.

By combining and/or sharing resources with fire and EMS departments, law enforcement agencies may be able to develop and implement more effective infection control programs. Law enforcement can use resources related to

- training and education issues
- cleaning and disinfecting facilities
- disposal facilities
- laundry areas
- protective clothing and equipment
- health maintenance
- joint infection control officer
- notification and verification of exposures relating an infectious disease

Fire and EMS departments can also provided guidance during the development and implementation of an infection control program, while tailoring the program to law enforcement needs.

Other Municipal/County Departments

Other municipal or county departments have the potential for possible exposure to airborne or bloodborne pathogens. Examples of departments or divisions that might be affected include, but are not limited to, medical examiner/coroner's office, social services, community mental health, general services (housekeeping), and sanitation. These departments also need an infection control program tailored to meet the needs of their specific duties and responsibilities relating to an exposure to a communicable disease. These departments may not have the expertise to develop a comprehensive infection control program and may need assistance from fire and EMS. Fire and EMS can provide direction, support, and share resources to ensure that members are adequately protected.

Vital issues for these departments can include

- training and education
- protective clothing and equipment
- health maintenance
- design of cleaning and disinfecting areas

- disposal areas

The most important factor is to ensure that proper control measures are in place in the event of an exposure. When providing medical care, regardless of the frequency and severity, the risk is still very real for any department's members.

SECTION 3
VEHICLES, EQUIPMENT, AND
SUPPLY CONSIDERATIONS

VEHICLES

All department vehicles involved in providing emergency medical services should comply with applicable and appropriate health and infection control laws, regulations, and standards. In addition, there are several factors that must be taken into consideration.

Vehicle operations pose many risks for a fire department and the firefighters that drive and ride on these vehicles. The operation of fire apparatus and vehicles during emergency and non-emergency response creates a liability for any fire department.

Another safety and health issue regarding vehicle safety relates to infection control procedures. As departments design new vehicles, consideration must be given to the ability to decontaminate the patient compartment and equipment. Other considerations, regarding infection control include ventilation, air filtration, and interior surfaces.

Emergency Vehicle Safety

An important component of the fire department's occupational safety and health program is vehicle operations. Vehicle operations encompass a wide spectrum of issues such as specifications, design, construction, purchase, operation, inspection, maintenance, response procedures, and repair of apparatus. In terms of member safety, a fully enclosed cab, seatbelts for all passengers, noise, warning lights and sirens, braking capacity, gross vehicle weight, infection control, and tool and equipment storage must be addressed during the initial specification phase.

Vehicles currently in use must be evaluated for risks and an action plan established to address and correct any safety issues. The HSO, the infection control officer, and the department's occupational safety and health committee must take a leading role to ensure the development and implementation of the action plan.

Ergonomics

The field of ergonomics studies methods used to perform a job task with the necessary tools and equipment and the physical skills used by an employee to perform that task. Any occupational task may be studied, but the focus is on repetitive tasks, particularly those that have resulted in numerous occupational injuries.

71

The fire service must incorporate ergonomics into the design of fire department vehicles and the use of tools and equipment. Before placing tools and equipment on vehicles, accessibility and the number of members needed to use them should be considered. Examples of ergonomics for tool and equipment placement include: backboards stored in compartments that allow removal without twisting or stretching, soft sleeves preconnected or stored near the inlet, traffic cones, and EMS equipment stored in a location for easy, frequent access.

When designing new vehicles, the placement and accessibility of tools and equipment are essential safety and ergonomics issues. As the design and use of enclosed fire apparatus continues, more and more tools and equipment are finding their way into the riding compartment. EMS equipment is being relocated to the interior for convenience, safety, and security. It is important to address the ability to remove equipment easily and safely without causing injury to firefighters (Figures 3-1 and 3-2).

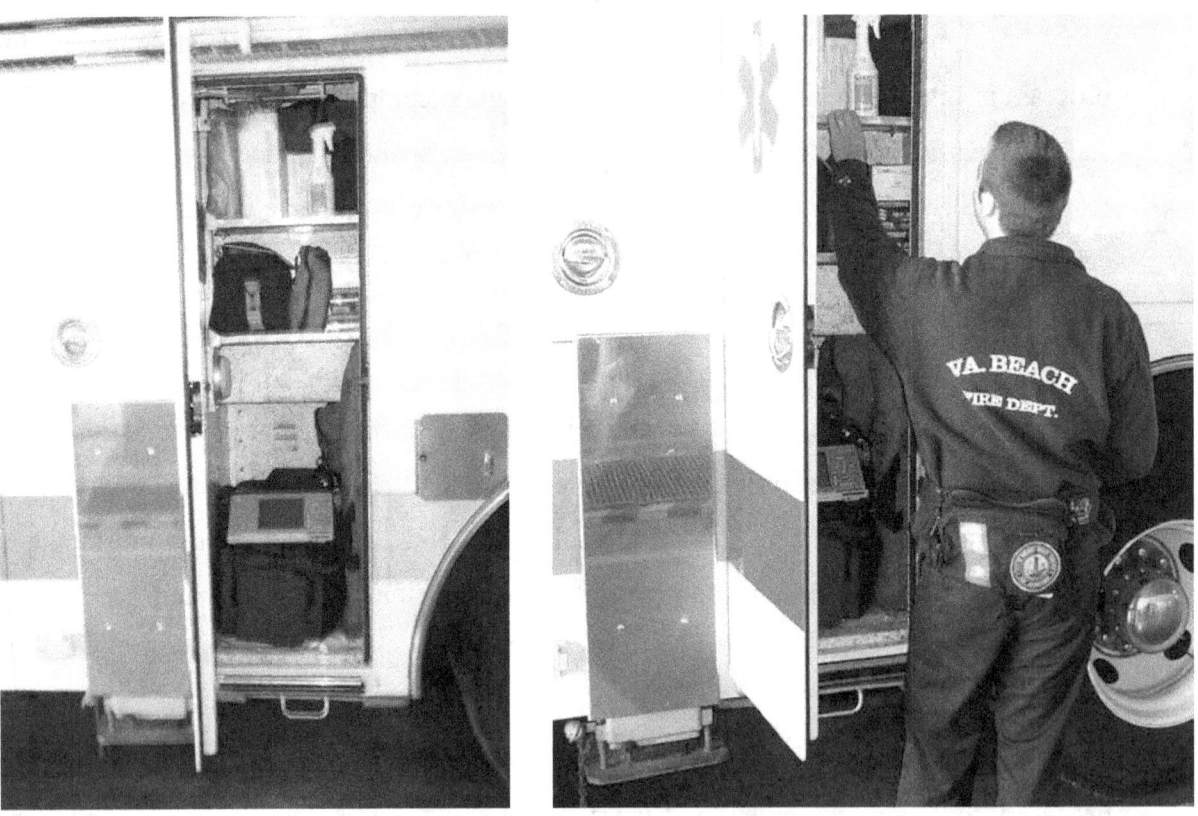

Figures 3-1 and 3-2 Equipment Placement
Photo courtesy of Murrey Loflin, Battalion Chief, Virginia Beach Fire Department

Fire Apparatus

Emergency medical services (EMS) equipment assigned to engine companies, truck companies, and rescue companies must be located in a designated compartment(s) on the apparatus. The compartments may need to be secured if Advanced Life Support medications are carried. Another safety and health consideration is the ability to clean and disinfect this compartment in the event of contamination from blood and body fluids. Although not as great an issue as on an ambulance, procedures must be in place in the event contaminated equipment is accidentally placed in the compartment.

In the event of an exposure to a member, procedures must be in place to decontaminate the member before he/she gets in or on the apparatus. An affected member may be placed in a disposable garment and transported back to quarters for proper cleaning. The personal protective equipment (PPE) must be placed in a biohazard bag and taken to quarters for evaluation for decontamination or disposal.

Ambulances

To ensure the safety of members operating and riding in an ambulance, the design and construction of the vehicle must meet appropriate design criteria such as those specified in the U.S. General Services Administration (GSA) Federal Specifications for the Star-of-Life Ambulance or KKK-A-1822 Specifications. This ensures that the steering, braking, seating capacity, patient care compartment, warning lights, electrical system, emergency medical care equipment, infection control, and other components are incorporated into the construction of the vehicle. The fire department must ensure that the vehicle is inspected prior to use and that regular preventive maintenance is performed per the manufacturer's guidelines.

NFPA 1500, *Standard on Fire Department Occupational Safety and Health Program*, requires that members performing emergency medical care must be secured to the vehicle by a seat belt or a safety harness while in an ambulance or rescue. The harness or belt is for the protection of the member providing medical care in the event of an accident, sudden stop, or start.

Design Considerations

As a fire department designs new vehicles used for patient care, strong consideration must be given to infection control. This is a prevention issue. Many problems can be avoided by effective planning and design of the interior of vehicles. The vehicle must be designed to meet the criteria established by applicable health and infection control laws, regulations, and standards - specifically criteria established by Occupational Safety and Health Administration (OSHA), Centers for Disease Control and Prevention (CDC), and the National Fire Protection Association (NFPA).

Vehicles that are used as rescue vehicles, ambulances, and non-emergency vehicles must comply with the guidelines, standards, and regulations established by these agencies. Engineering controls will enhance the infection control process when used with training, effective infection control practices, appropriate personal protective clothing and equipment, and disinfecting and cleaning procedures.

The ventilation of an ambulance is critical for the safety and health of members operating inside the vehicle. NFPA 1581 includes the following criteria for adequate and effective ventilation. The ventilation system must provide complete ambient air exchange in both the driver and patient compartments on a regular basis. Control of the ventilation system should be possible from both compartments. Fresh air intakes should be located towards the front of the vehicle to afford maximum intake of fresh air. Exhaust vents should be located in the upper rear of the vehicle. To reduce the risk of tuberculosis, high efficiency particulate arresting (HEPA) filters should be integrated in the patient compartment ventilation system. All seats, mounted cushions, cots, floors, counters, shelves, bulkheads, and container linings must be made of or covered by non-absorbent, washable material. These surface materials should be inert to detergents, solutions, and solvents, for disinfecting and cleaning as described by OSHA or CDC. Some simple design considerations for an ambulance regarding ventilation are

- When a vehicle is stationary, the ventilation systems shall provide complete exchange of ambient air in both the driver and patient compartment every 2 minutes.

- Fresh air intakes for the ventilation shall be located towards the front of the vehicle.

- Exhaust systems should be located on the upper rear of the vehicle.

- Ventilation for the patient compartment shall be separate from the power intake or exhaust ventilation system.

- Interior surfaces must be covered by or comprised of nonabsorbent, washable material.

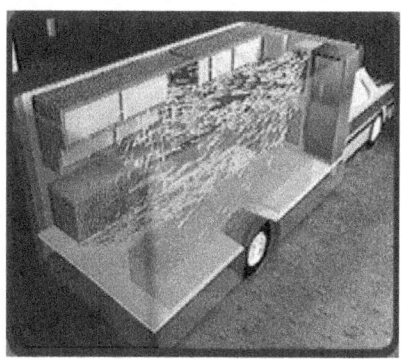

Figure 3-3 Ambulance Air Filtration
Photo Courtesy of Wheeled Coach

There are now transport units available with self-contained purification units that exchange patient compartment air in less than 90 seconds and remove particles 0.3 microns and larger at 99.97 percent efficiency. (See Figure 3-3.)

Decontamination and Disinfection of Vehicles

The fire department must consider engineering controls for proper decontamination and disinfecting when designing new vehicles and apparatus. EMS compartments on fire apparatus and other vehicles should be designed to facilitate easy decontamination and disinfecting in the event contaminated materials are placed in these compartments.

All disinfectants used should be approved and registered with the Environmental Protection Agency (EPA) as tuberculocidal. If a disinfectant is tuberculocidal, it is strong enough to kill all other bacteria and virus of concern. Members using disinfectants must be aware of safety and health precautions such as ventilation, use of appropriate PPE, and flammability and reactivity of the disinfectants. A chlorine bleach solution also can be used to disinfect compartments, hard surfaces, or other areas of a vehicle or apparatus. The CDC's *Recommendations for Prevention of HIV Transmission in Health-Care Settings* (MMWR, 39:RR17) states that effective concentrations range from 500 ppm (1:100) to 5,000 ppm (1:10) depending on the amount of organic material present on the surface. Surfaces first should be washed with hot soapy water and then rinsed with clean water so all visible material has been removed. If organic material has been removed by cleaning, the lower concentration of bleach (1:100) appears to be effective. A 1:100 dilution can be attained by mixing approximately 2 cups of chlorine bleach per gallon of water. The lower concentration is preferable whenever possible since stronger concentrations may corrode or destroy vulnerable metal with continued use. The bleach solution should be prepared daily. Use of commercial disinfectants should follow manufacturers' instructions.

PERSONAL PROTECTIVE EQUIPMENT

Hand washing and effective personal hygiene are key factors in reducing the risk of contracting a communicable disease. If hand washing is not feasible, antiseptic soap (waterless) or wipes should be used. Hands should be washed immediately after PPE is removed. Hands, mucous membranes, or exposed skin should be washed after an exposure to blood or body fluids.

PPE serves as a control measure to reduce the risk of an exposure. The purpose of PPE is to provide a barrier to prevent personal contact with blood or other potentially infectious materials. PPE includes gloves, masks, protective eyewear, and gowns; it must be provided at no cost to the employee. Some departments issue waist or "fanny" packs for carrying PPE (Figure 3-4).

The potential risk of an exposure determines the type of PPE used. The minimum PPE used should be examination gloves. The greater the risk of an exposure to blood or body fluids, the more protective clothing should be used. Due to health problems resulting from latex examination gloves, the employer must provide a variety of hypoallergenic gloves in a variety of sizes. Structural firefighting protective clothing serves as an excellent barrier against blood and body fluids. When firefighters are performing vehicle extrication, turnout gear (helmet, coat, pants, boots, and gloves) is the optimum choice of PPE to prevent injuries/exposures from sharp surfaces or obstructions.

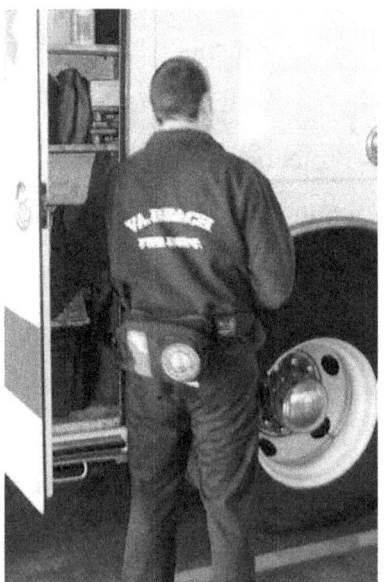

Figure 3-4 "Fanny" Pack
Photo courtesy of Murrey Loflin, Battalion Chief, Virginia Beach Fire Department, Virginia Beach, VA.

Gloves

Members providing emergency medical care must don emergency medical gloves. Medical gloves are single-use, designed to provide barrier protection against body fluids while examining and caring for patients. Medical gloves are a standard component of emergency medical response equipment. Latex-free gloves must be provided for members with a latex allergy or for use when providing medical care to patients with a latex allergy.

Emergency medical gloves should be removed as soon as possible after the completion of patient care. Care must be taken to prevent skin contact with the gloves' surface, and they should be properly disposed of per the department's SOP.

Vinyl or latex gloves specifically recommended for patient care should be used on all responses where there is any potential for exposure to blood or body fluids. Providers should put on gloves **before** contact with the patient. It is not an uncommon practice for providers to don gloves enroute, based on dispatch information.

Gloves that become grossly contaminated, punctured, or torn at the scene should be changed as soon as it can be done safely. Hands should be washed before donning new gloves. A waterless hand cleaner should be used if normal hand washing facilities are not available at the scene. Double gloving may also be considered when providers are in situations with a large amount of blood/body fluids, when there is a potential for gloves being torn or punctured by the surrounding environment, or when dealing with multiple patients.

Heavy gloves, such as structural firefighting gloves, should be used for extricating a patient and where broken glass or jagged metal is present. Since these gloves do not provide a moisture barrier, vinyl or latex gloves should be worn under them. Structural firefighting gloves, if available, should be worn where sharp or rough surfaces or potentially high heat exposure may be encountered, such as vehicle extrication. Medical gloves should not be worn under structural firefighting gloves when there is potential for exposure to heat. Heat can cause the emergency medical glove to burn, melt, or drip. Structural firefighting gloves that become contaminated should be disinfected and cleaned per manufacturer's instructions. The vinyl or latex gloves used for patient contact also are not adequate for cleaning soiled equipment or vehicles. These tasks require a more durable glove.

About 10 percent of health-care workers are allergic to latex.[5] The infection control officer should work with the department medical director to determine appropriate gloves made of other materials for use by any provider who is allergic to latex.

Masks

Masks (and protective eyewear) should be used during situations involving excessive exposure to blood, trauma, childbirth, and other situations where gross contamination is anticipated or encountered. Masks are designed to limit exposure of the nasal, oral, respiratory, or mucosal membranes to bloodborne and airborne pathogens.

Surgical masks (Figure 3-5) are designed to prevent **blood** or **body fluids** from coming in contact with the mouth and nose. These are disposable, single-use masks. Some surgical masks are designed with a face shield attached. They do not protect against airborne pathogens such as tuberculosis.

A NIOSH-approved, N-95 or HEPA respirator (Figure 3-6) should be worn the entire time a provider is in contact with a patient suspected of having tuberculosis. If the patient is not suffering any respiratory distress, placing a surgical mask on the patient will reduce the release of droplets from coughing.

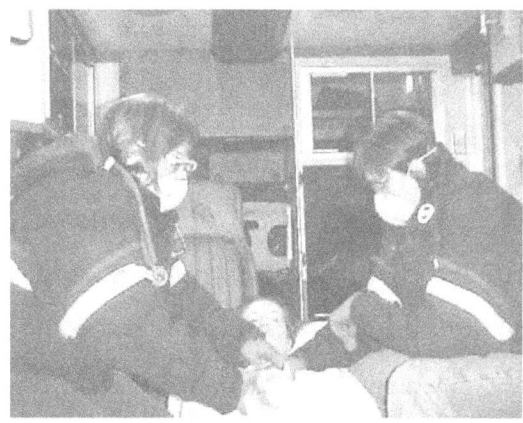

Figure 3-5 Standard Surgical Mask

Photo courtesy of Fairfield Fire & EMS,
Fairfield. PA

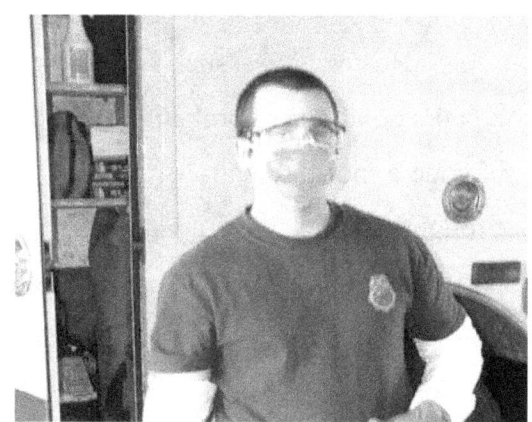

Figure 3-6 HEPA Mask

Photo courtesy of Murrey Loflin, Battalion
Chief, Virginia Beach Fire Department,
Virginia Beach, VA

Eye Protection

Protective eyewear should be donned in any situation with the potential for blood or body fluids to come in contact with the eyes. Acceptable eye protection includes goggles or glasses with side protectors. Providers who normally wear glasses can have them modified with clip-on side protectors or use goggles designed to be worn over the glasses. Providers should remember that touching the eyes while wearing potentially contaminated gloves should be avoided. Figure 3-7 shows protective eyewear with side protectors.

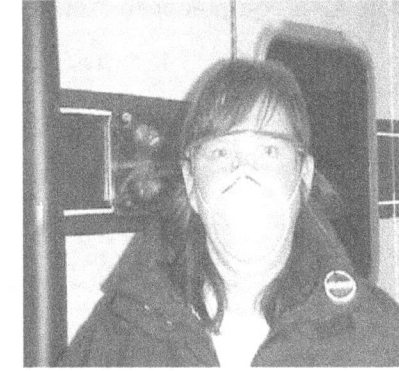

Figure 3-7 Protective Eyewear
Photo Courtesy of Fairfield Fire & EMS

Gowns

Gowns should be worn to provide a barrier to blood/body fluid in situations where heavy bleeding may contaminate clothing, including childbirth. Gowns should also be worn while cleaning the vehicle after a response if it is heavily contaminated by blood. Table 3-1 summarizes which type of PPE is indicated in specific situations.

Table 3-1 When and Which Types of Person Protective Equipment to Use				
Activity	**Gloves**	**Eyewear**	**Mask**	**Gown**
Uncontrolled bleeding	Yes	Yes	Yes	Yes
Controlled bleeding	Yes	No	No	No
Childbirth	Yes	Yes	Yes	Yes
Endotracheal intubation	Yes	Yes	Yes	No
Oral/Nasal suctioning, manually cleaning airway	Yes	Yes	Yes	Yes
Handling/Cleaning possibly contaminated instruments	Yes	Yes	Yes	Yes
Measuring blood pressure	No*	No	No	No
Giving an injection/Starting an IV	Yes	No	No	No
Measuring temperature	Yes	No	No	No
Cleaning patient compartment after a call	Yes	No**	No**	No**

* Unless the patient's arm is contaminated with blood or body fluids or unless required by department policy.

** Unless heavily contaminated by blood or body fluids or unless required by department policy.

Dickinson, E. (1999). *Fire Service Emergency Care*. Upper Saddle River, NJ; Prentice-Hall, Inc. Reprinted with permission.

Sleeves

Sleeves provide protection of exposed skin of the arms. Sleeves are valuable personal protective equipment for services operating in warm climates and when long-sleeved apparel is not worn. Figure 3-8 shows the use of protective sleeves.

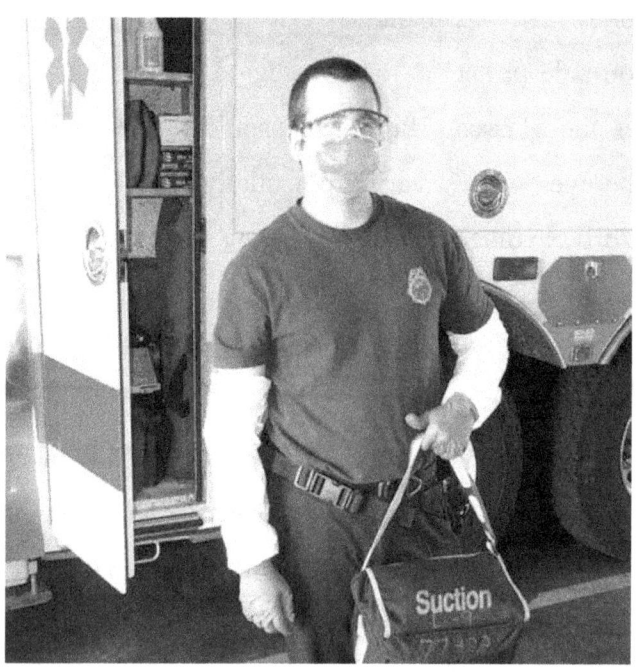

Figure 3-8 Protective Sleeves
Photo courtesy of Murrey Loflin, Battalion Chief, Virginia Beach Fire Department, Virginia Beach, VA

PPE should be cleaned, washed/laundered, or disposed of appropriately by the employer at no cost to the worker. All PPE should remain at the worksite. If at all possible, nothing should be taken home in order to prevent cross-contamination of family clothing. Contaminated PPE that can be decontaminated and cleaned can be reused. If cleaning and decontamination is not possible, the equipment must be disposed of properly in an approved method. Laundering provisions located in fire stations need to be separate from the laundering equipment used for normal cleaning such as linens, uniforms, and towels. The hot water must be above 130 degrees, and waste water must empty into a sanitary sewer system.

EQUIPMENT AND SUPPLIES

Biohazardous Waste Disposal

Many of the items used for patient care, such as bag-valve-masks (BVM), suction catheters, etc., are single-use, disposable and should be properly disposed of after use. Some items, such as bag-valve-masks (BVM), may be left with the patient at the hospital for continued use, unless they are grossly contaminated.

Grossly contaminated BVM's and other single-use items, with the exception of needles, must be placed in a red bag or container marked with a biohazard seal (Figure 3-9). Needles and other sharp objects should be placed in a puncture-proof container that is designated for biohazard waste disposal. Disposal of biohazardous waste should follow the department's written procedure.

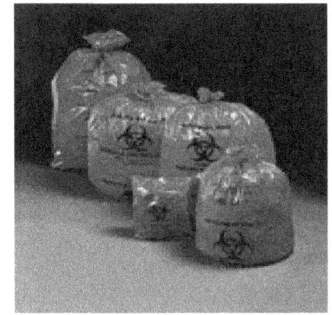

Figure 3-9. Biohazard Bag

Non-Disposable Equipment

Surfaces of non-disposable equipment that may have come in contact with a patient's blood or body fluids must be cleaned, disinfected, or sterilized. Non-disposable equipment includes blood pressure cuffs, splints, backboards, cervical immobilization devices, laryngoscope blades, etc. Cleaning means washing the item with soap and water. Disinfecting involves the use of a disinfectant that kills some microorganisms. Sterilization, either chemical or superheated steam in an autoclave, kills all microorganisms.

Equipment in Contact with Intact Skin

In the majority of patient contacts, the blood pressure cuff and stethoscope are in contact with intact skin. In many instances, splints, backboards, and cervical immobilization devices contact only intact skin. For equipment that contacts only intact skin, cleaning and disinfecting with a 1:100 bleach solution or EPA-registered tuberculocidal disinfectant is adequate. These disinfectants will destroy mycobacterium tuberculosis, most viruses, vegetative bacteria, and most fungi.

Equipment in Contact with Mucous Membranes

Equipment such as laryngoscopes, blades, and handles that come in contact with mucous membranes should be either chemically sterilized with an EPA-registered chemical sterilant for 10 to 45 minutes after cleaning, or autoclaved. The chemical sterilant will destroy mycobacterium tuberculosis, most viruses, vegetative bacteria, and most fungi. Many services leave the used equipment at the hospital for sterilization and replace it with new equipment from hospital stock.

Equipment Contaminated with Blood/Body Fluids

Any equipment contaminated with blood or body fluids first should be cleaned of all visible material since disinfectants are less effective when they must penetrate dirt and other debris. Gloves that are heavy enough to resist puncture from sharp edges should be worn while cleaning the equipment. If there is a potential for splashing, face protection, eyewear, and fluid- impervious gown or apron also should be used. Disposable towels should be used if available. If disposable towels are not available, use towels that can be placed in a plastic bag for contaminated laundry after the cleaning is complete.

Following cleaning, the equipment should be decontaminated with a germicide following manufacturer's instructions or a 1:100 bleach solution using clean towels. All equipment should be allowed to air dry. After decontamination is complete, place gloves in a sealed plastic bag for disposal and wash hands.

EQUIPMENT ADVANCES
Backboards

Backboards are now available made of material that is resistant to penetration by body fluids and chemicals, thus are easier to clean and disinfect. Figure 3-10 is an example of one of these plastic backboards.

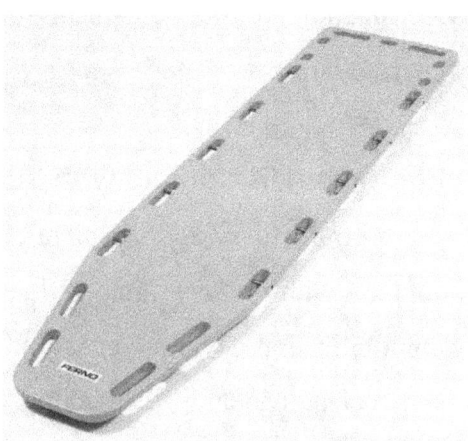

Figure 3-10. Plastic Backboard
Photo courtesy of Ferno

Cervical Immobilization Devices

Cervical Immobilization Devices (CID) are available in both disposable and non-disposable forms (Figures 3-11 and 3-12). Most disposable CID's are corrugated material that is treated to be water-resistant. The disposable CID's have some limitations, but may be an option for mass casualties. Non-disposable CID's also are water-proofed with smooth surfaces that make cleaning easier.

Although this new construction assists in the ease of cleaning and decontaminating, care must be taken to assure that the Velcro straps used to immobilize patients to the backboard and to assure placement of CID's are also cleaned and decontaminated appropriately.

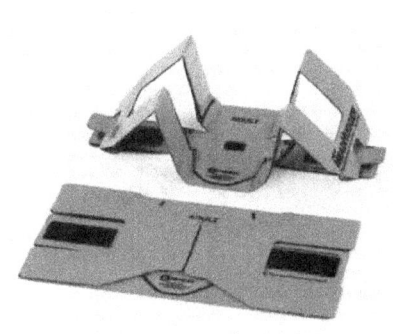

Figure 3-11. Disposable CID
Photo courtesy of Ferno

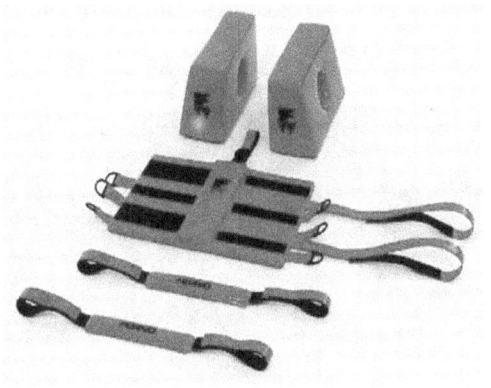

Figure 3-12. Non-disposable CID
Photo courtesy of Ferno

Needleless Systems

The most common bloodborne pathogen exposure is the needlestick that results while recapping a needle. This particular cause of needlesticks should be totally preventable. As a result of changes in technology, there is a renewed strong focus on reducing needlestick injuries. In 1999, several legislative initiatives and regulatory agencies began the process of addressing changes to decrease the potential for infectious diseases as the result of needlesticks. The Health Care Worker Needlestick Safety and Prevention Act was signed into law in November 2000. Sixteen States have already passed needle safety legislation and it is pending in one other State. Table 3-2 summarizes the States that have passed needle safety legislation to date.

Table 3-2   **States with Needle Safety Legislation**

California	Maryland	Oklahoma
Alaska	Massachusetts	Tennessee
Connecticut	Minnesota	Texas
Georgia	New Hampshire	West Virginia
Iowa	New Jersey	Pennsylvania (pending)
Maine	Ohio	

Revisions to the *Occupational Exposure to Bloodborne Pathogens* (29 CFR Part 1910.1030) obligate employers to consider safer needle devices when they conduct their annual review of their exposure control plan and requires that a log of injuries from contaminated sharps be maintained.

An increasing number and variety of needle devices with safety features are now available. Figure 3-13 is an example of one of these devices. This needleless system has a built-in flow valve that helps prevent blood exposure.

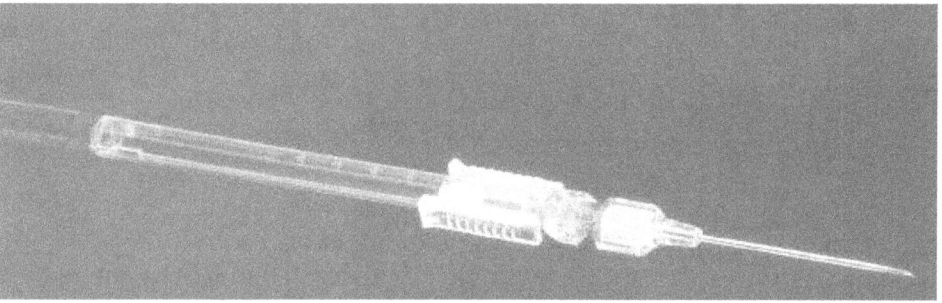

Figure 3-13. Secure IV™ Needleless System
Photo courtesy of Vadus

Because of the proliferation of needle devices with safety features, many of these devices have had only limited use in the workplace. As a result, NIOSH released its Alert: Preventing Needlestick Injuries in Health Care Settings, which states that needle devices with safety features should be evaluated to ensure that:

- the safety feature works effectively and reliably
- the device is acceptable to the health care worker
- the device does not adversely affect patient care

As EMS services evaluate needleless systems, consider cost of the devices and resupply issues. If the service resupplies these items on an exchange system with the local hospital(s), it would be in the best interest of the EMS service program to work with the hospitals in the evaluation process to determine which needle device will be used. Even if the service does not obtain resupply from area hospitals, those hospitals should be contacted to gather information from their evaluations of, and experience with, different types of devices.

Waterless Hand Cleaners

As stated earlier in this manual, hand washing with regular soap and water is the most important method of preventing the spread of infectious diseases. Hands should be washed after each patient encounter, after all cleaning and decontamination of equipment, and immediately after each contact with a potentially contaminated patient or item. There are several occasions when hand washing is desirable, but there is no water available. Examples include a patient refusal when the provider removes his/her gloves, or when patient care requires a glove change due to a tear. When water is unavailable, there are several commercial waterless hand cleaners available for use. Waterless cleaners come in both gel or wipe form. The main ingredient in the waterless cleansers is alcohol. Several brands also contain PCMX, a manmade phenolic active (antiseptic compound).

OTHER CONSIDERATIONS
Clothing and Linen

Although the risk of disease transmission from soiled clothing or linen is minimal, the risk should not be ignored. There are several steps that the provider should take to reduce the risk.

Dirty clothes should be changed as soon as possible and the provider should shower before donning clean clothes. Providers should keep at least one extra uniform at the station while on duty. Volunteers who respond from home should keep an extra change of clothes at the station for use if needed when returning from a call, or carry an extra set in their vehicle.

Dirty linen and clothing should be handled as little as possible. Soiled items should be bagged, with blood-contaminated clothing/linen placed in a separate, leak-proof bag marked with a biohazard label. Soiled clothing/linen should be washed in the normal laundry cycles with regular detergent following label instructions. Gloves should be used when handling, bagging, and placing dirty items in the washing machine.

If a volunteer provider's clothes are contaminated with blood or body fluid, it should be a policy that he/she return to the station to shower, change, and bag the soiled clothing in a controlled environment rather than driving home directly following a call. It is preferable that the contaminated clothing be washed at the station. If laundry facilities are not available at the station, the department must make alternative arrangements for laundering so contaminated items are not taken home. This may include arrangements with other departments, hospitals, or commercial laundry facilities.

Responding From/Returning to Home or Work

Volunteers who respond from and return to home or the primary work site have an obligation to protect patients and the public from the potential of infectious disease as well as protecting themselves. The issue of contaminated clothing for volunteers returning home from a call has been addressed above. What must also be considered is the workplace environment and conditions when the volunteer responds. If the work environment (e.g., working around animals, food handling of raw meat, construction work, etc.) carries the possibility of disease-causing germs to be present, the provider must take the time to wash hands thoroughly and be sure clothes are not soiled before responding and coming in contact with the patient. The same holds true if the potential exists to transmit disease from the patient to co-workers on return to the primary job.

Since volunteers may respond to the scene in a private vehicle to render care while waiting for the ambulance, it is important to be careful that blood or body fluids are not carried back to the interior of the personal vehicle. It also may be a reasonable policy to supply personnel who do not accompany the patient during transport with waterless hand cleaner to use before re-entering their private vehicle to return to work.

Resource Management

Although a rare occurrence, service programs should have a plan in place to access additional infection control supplies on short notice in situations such as mass casualty incidents that may deplete the normal supply level rapidly. Access to other service programs' supplies through mutual-aid agreements may handle the extra demand. Other options include having an emergency number for a local vendor or developing an agreement with the local hospital(s) to get an emergency stock if needed.

SUMMARY

OSHA regulations, CDC guidelines, and NFPA standards have affected the operations and management of emergency service agencies. The intent of these regulations and standards is to provide protection for employees at risk for an exposure to blood or body fluids.

Occupationally, an exposure to a communicable disease can have devastating results for members. Contracting a communicable disease could lead to death, long-term disability, early retirement, significant health concerns, and reduced life expectancy. It is critical that following an exposure, the member be seen for medical follow-up as soon as possible. Optimal use of post exposure prophylaxis (PEP) for HIV requires treatment within hours.

Infection control must become a significant part of the daily operations of emergency responders. The delivery of emergency medical services continues to be a major part of service delivery for fire departments. The potential for an exposure is an occupational risk that emergency service personnel face every day.

This chapter discussed many ways to reduce and eliminate exposures to airborne and bloodborne diseases. Members must realize that this is a real occupational threat. The cost of treating an exposure is momentous, and can have a major financial impact on the department. Moreover, the human side has more cataclysmic results that affect the individual, family, department, and community. The exposure to blood or body fluids is truly an occupational hazard that must be addressed properly as part of a department's occupational safety and health program. As a department develops or revises its mission statement, infection control should become a vital part of the process.

SECTION 4

FACILITY CONSIDERATIONS

THE NEED FOR FACILITY SAFETY

A successful occupational safety and health program must address facility safety, which encompasses fire stations, offices, shop areas, and any other area where personnel work while on duty. NFPA 1500, *Standard on Fire Department Occupational Safety and Health Program*, defines a fire department facility as

> Any building or area owned, operated, occupied, or used by a fire department on a routine basis. This does not include locations where a fire department can be summoned to perform emergency operations or other duties, unless such premises are normally under the control of the fire department.

Most firefighters' duties and activities focus around the fire station. The majority of on-duty time is spent in fire stations, training centers, administrative offices, and department shop areas. The facility environment must be routinely examined to ensure the safety of the personnel. Hazards and unsafe conditions that exist in the fire station or in other fire department facilities can endanger both personnel and visitors who enter these facilities.

The design, construction, maintenance, and general upkeep of fire department facilities are a major financial expense. Depending on the funding, operation, and composition of a fire department, the facilities may be used for a variety of functions. One building may house multiple functions including an assembly area for meetings or other social functions, administrative offices, apparatus repair/shop, training center, dispatch center, and fire station.

NFPA 1500 requires the Health and Safety Officer (HSO) to ensure that all facilities are inspected at least annually to assure the safest working environment possible. Personnel assigned to these facilities must take responsibility to correct any unsafe condition by conducting at least a monthly inspection. If unsafe conditions are found, procedures must be in place to correct any hazards or code violations and to prevent an accident or possible injury.

Infection Control

Fire department facilities are not exempt from regulations and standards that address a safe and healthy work environment. Facilities must be designed to provide the proper working conditions and conform to infection control standards. Proper equipment, protective clothing, and disposal of infectious waste must be provided to ensure compliance with *Occupational Exposure to Bloodborne Pathogens* (29 CFR Part 1910.1030). If emergency medical care is provided by the department, the facility will need to be equipped with a decontamination area to clean and disinfect personnel, protective clothing, and equipment properly. An excellent resource for guidance in developing a fire department infection control program is NFPA 1581, *Standard on Fire Department Infection Control Program.*

Facility safety and health is just one part of the infection control process. Infection control procedures should address issues such as:

- Hand washing
- Need for protective clothing and equipment while disinfecting and cleaning
- How to properly and effectively disinfect medical equipment, protective clothing, and protective equipment
- Disinfecting and cleaning areas once finished
- Proper disposal of contaminated materials in a container marked infectious waste
- Proper storage and disposal of sharps in a sharps container

Adherence to all State and local laws governing infection control and compliance is required. Failure to comply with these regulations can cause an occupational exposure and create added liability for the fire department. Alan Brunacini, Fire Chief of the Phoenix Fire Department, summarized the importance of complying with regulations when he said, "Safety prevents meetings."[5] Compliance is a less expensive method.

---

[5] Brunacini, A. (1985). *Fire command.* National Fire Protection Association; College Park, MD: YBS Productions; p. 244.

Decontamination Areas

Decontamination needs to be carried out in separate areas that are properly marked and secured. Appropriate disinfecting supplies must be available. A nonporous sink, such as stainless steel, with hot and cold running water, should be available. Nonporous materials are safer than traditional porous materials such as wood, plastic, and porcelain. Porous materials have a tendency to allow foreign matter to permeate the surface, which makes disinfecting the sink difficult. Other equipment needed for the decontamination area includes

- Racks or shelves for air-drying of equipment
- Two sinks
- Sprayer attachment
- Drains attached to sanitary sewer system or septic system
- Faucets that are turned on by elbow, foot, or sensor (Figure 4-1)
- Continuous molded counter tops/splash panels
- Proper lighting
- Proper ventilation
- Floor drains attached to the sanitary sewer system

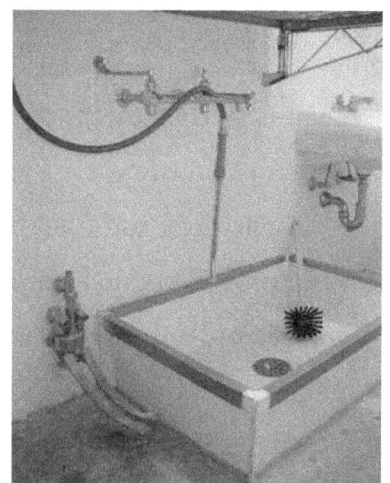

Figure 4-1 Sink with foot controls.
Photo Courtesy of Steve Weissman, Captain Fairfax County Fire, Fairfax, VA.

Most fire stations were not initially designed to incorporate decontamination of infectious waste. This need surfaced in the early 1990's. Fire stations that do not have a separate or available room for decontamination may have to add a room or a separate building. Decontamination of personnel and cleaning and disinfecting equipment must never be done in the kitchen, living, sleeping, or personal hygiene areas.

FACILITY ISSUES

Each area of a fire station or fire department facility has particular safety and health issues and features that need to be identified, evaluated, implemented, and monitored.

Kitchen

The kitchen is the central location of activities in most fire stations. Activities routinely occurring in the kitchen include food preparation, eating, discussions/meetings, and watching television. With so many activities occurring in this area, safety and health procedures are paramount. **Medical equipment should never be cleaned, disinfected, or stored in the kitchen area.** All equipment cleaning should be done in a designated area to prevent chemical or biological agents from coming in contact with food and food preparation utensils and equipment.

Double sinks and a dishwasher should be provided to clean dishes and utensils properly. The refrigerator/freezer should maintain foods at proper temperatures -- cold storage 38° F (3° C) or less, and freezer temperatures at 0° F (-18° C) or less. In addition to regular inspections, a thermometer should be placed in a conspicuous place in both the refrigerator and the freezer.

Countertops and shelving should be constructed of nonporous materials. Food should be properly heated to kill the parasites or bacteria and leftovers should be covered for storage. In the event of an alarm, food should be stored properly to prevent food poisoning.

All members working in the kitchen must use good safety practices. Common safety practices include

- Cleaning up after spills
- Storing sharp objects, especially knives, in a safe manner
- Discouraging horseplay
- Watching food on the stove at all times
- Promptly turning off all burners and ovens when not in use
- Using all appliances in accordance with manufacturer's instructions
- Exercising extreme caution when using knives, graters, slicers, or can openers

Sleeping Quarters

According to NFPA 1581, there should be a minimum of 60 square feet of floor space for each bed space in sleeping areas. This provides rapid and easy access during alarms. The required floor space per bed also is designed to reduce the chances of spreading colds or other airborne diseases among members, and to make sleep easier.

Separate bedding and clothing lockers should be provided for each member who requires a bed. Proper ventilation, heating, and cooling are essential to the health of personnel living in the fire station. Sleeping quarters should be separated by a 1-hour fire-resistive wall and be equipped with a smoke detector(s), a carbon monoxide detector, and a sprinkler system.

Bathrooms

Personal hygiene is a fundamental defense against preventing illness and communicable diseases. All fire department facilities should have the proper facilities for washing and cleaning. Hand washing should be done only in restrooms or bathrooms, not in the kitchen.

Restrooms and bathrooms can be a significant source of infection if they are poorly designed and maintained. They must be kept sanitary. Bathrooms should have push-to-open doors for egress. This eliminates a place for infectious agents to accumulate and breed. It should not be necessary for members to grip sink controls in order to turn them on or off. If the handle must be grasped, a paper towel should be used to turn it off after drying. Hand drying materials should be disposable, or an air-drying machine should be available. Use of a cloth or towel presents the potential for infectious agents to accumulate. There is minimal potential of bacteria being on disposable hand drying material, so it can be disposed of like regular household refuse.

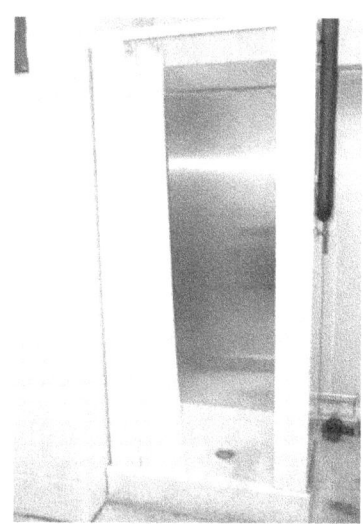

Figure 4-2 Shower curtain to minimize water reaching the floor.

Photo courtesy of Murrey Loflin, Battalion Chief. Virginia Beach Fire

Showers should be cleaned regularly to prevent the growth of mold and mildew. Showers should have curtains or doors to minimize the amount of water that reaches the floor (Figure 4-2). Safety glass or plastic panels should be used in the shower doors. Drying racks for towels should be available, as well as good ventilation to prevent mold and mildew. The flush valves on toilets and urinals should be foot-operated or use an electric eye so hands are not required to operate it. Most importantly, a clear and visible sign should be mounted prominently in each bathroom to remind members to wash their hands.

Storage

Clean equipment and unused supplies should have a separate storage area. This ensures that contaminants are isolated. The storage area needs to be conspicuously marked and secured. In the event a separate area is not available, a secure locker or cabinet can be used as a suitable substitute.

General storage areas have a tendency to become disorganized and cluttered, which can cause slips, falls, fire, or injury from a falling object. Some general safety considerations should be

- Limiting storage in utility rooms
- Assuring storage is well organized and maintained
- Storing heavy items near the floor
- Assuring no items block utility boxes or escapes
- Storing flammable liquids in safety containers
- Storing containers for flammable liquids away from heat sources, preferably in a storage container or outside the facility
- Properly marking containers' contents

Laundry Areas

The fire department should provide a designated area equipped with a washer and dryer in each fire station for cleaning station work uniforms, protective clothing, and linens (Figure 4-3). All necessary detergents and prescrub, proper water temperature, and laundering instructions should be available. This eliminates the need for members to take contaminated uniforms or clothing home, which might cross-contaminate the family laundry.

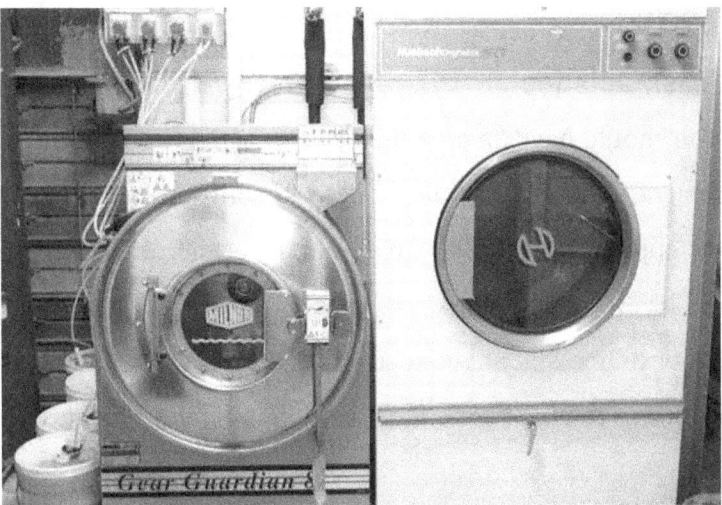

Figure 4-3. Fire station washer and dryer prevent cross-contamination to family laundry.
Photo courtesy of Murrey Loflin, Battalion Chief, Virginia Beach Fire Department, Virginia Beach , VA.

To comply with these requirements, most fire departments have provided the following:

- At least one washer and dryer in the station for laundering station work uniforms

- A laundry service for station work uniforms and protective clothing

- A centrally located commercial washer and dryer for laundering protective clothing

The laundry area should also provide a means for cleaning and other laundry items in a washer and dryer that is used only for non-contaminated items. For contaminated items, a commercial washer and dryer must be provided, or a laundry service contracted for proper cleaning and decontamination.

Cleaning Areas

Similar to the laundry area, a designated cleaning area must be provided for cleaning personal protective equipment (PPE), portable equipment, and any other contaminated clothing and equipment. The cleaning areas must have proper ventilation, lighting, and drainage connected to a sanitary sewer or a septic system. This area must be separate from the areas used for food preparation, eating, sleeping, living areas, and personal hygiene. This area must also be separate from the disinfecting area.

Disinfecting Areas/Facilities

A fire station should have an area that is designated for disinfecting contaminated clothing and equipment. This area should be accessible from the outside of the facility as well as through the apparatus bay. The area must meet the requirements established by the local and State health departments. It must be equipped with proper lighting and ventilation, have floor drains that are connected to a sanitary sewer or septic system, and be properly maintained in terms of general housekeeping requirements.

Disposal Areas

Effective cleaning and disinfecting areas include a method for proper disposal of contaminated waste. Disposal shall take place in a properly marked and secured area separate from the kitchen, living, personal hygiene, and sleeping areas. Disposal of infectious waste must meet State and local laws and regulations pertaining to the handling, storage, transportation, and disposal of medical or infectious waste. Proper containers must be marked and used for disposal purposes, and not used for the disposal of regular waste or trash.

SUMMARY

Whether a department is designing a new facility or renovating a current facility, the most important factor is infection control. Financial obligations from the governing entity will need to be considered in order to bring a facility into compliance with the applicable and appropriate health and infection control laws, codes, and standards for fire department or EMS facilities. Prevention is much more cost effective than having to pay workers' compensation claims resulting from exposures to an infectious disease. The U.S. Fire Administration's *Safety and Health Considerations for the Design of Fire and Emergency Medical Services Stations* (1997) provides a comprehensive resource for other facility design considerations.

SECTION 5

ASSESSING EFFECTIVENESS: THE EVALUATION PROCESS

OVERVIEW

Any program is incomplete without a formal evaluation process. Managing any program is best described as an ongoing cyclical process (Figure 5-1).

Figure 5-1

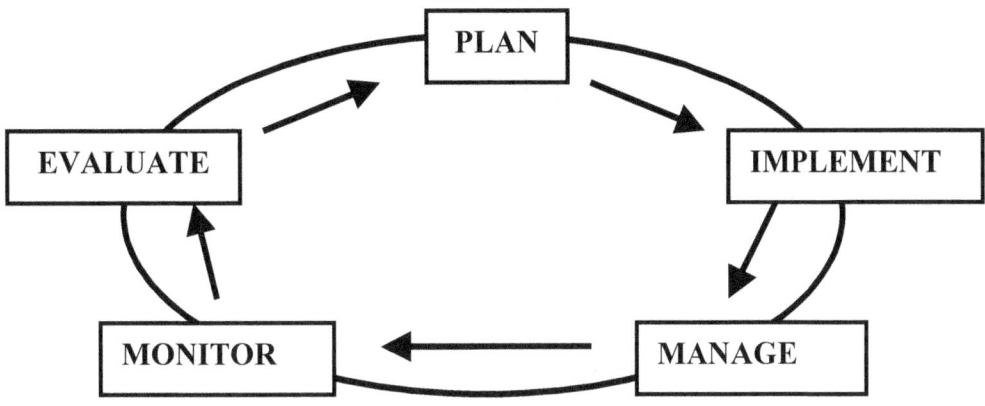

Thus, although evaluation is the "final" step, it actually leads to a repetition of the development cycle.

Evaluation is a systematic analysis of program activities and results for the purpose of determining the program's overall effectiveness. The evaluation process should address two specific aspects: 1) compliance with the performance indicators of the existing program, and 2) the attainment of the program goal. Quality monitoring is used to determine whether individuals in the organization are complying with established protocols/performance standards. In other words, quality monitoring answers the question: Are we doing things right? Program evaluation answers the question: Are we doing the right things?

Program analysis relies on a systematic analysis of various types of data collected over a predetermined period of time. The focus is on identifying measurable **changes** that have occurred as a result of the program. Data collected from quality monitoring is one source of information used to determine if the program is meeting the overall program goal. Review of changes in laws and standards and changes in technology also should be used to determine if the program is accomplishing what it should. Analysis of these data should be used to identify what needs to be done to improve program effectiveness. In effect, this leads back to the planning component.

ASSESSING EFFECTIVENESS

In very simple terms, the evaluation phase focuses on measuring the difference between what was happening before and what is happening now. In order to compare the differences, evaluation criteria/performance indicators must be written in measurable terms with an expected outcome stated (compliance level). Performance indicators should be reviewed and revised on a regular basis. By analyzing data on a regular basis, the organization will be able to revise performance indicators based on compliance, new technology, or changing laws/regulations. Performance indicators should be based on governmental regulations, such as Occupational Safety and Health Administration (OSHA), and national standards, such as National Fire Protection Association (NFPA) 1500 and NFPA 1581.

Developing Objectives and Performance Indicators
Objectives

Performance indicators are developed from the objectives identified for the program. The objectives should be defined during the planning (or revision) phase of the program management cycle and should be consistent with the goal of the organization -- injury prevention and preventive health care. Objectives should be

- S – specific
- M – measurable
- A – attainable
- R – realistic
- T – timely

Some objectives, when well-defined, also can be used as performance indicators. However, other objectives may be too broad to use as performance indicators. For example: an organization has documented 40 accidental needlesticks during IV initiation (4% of all IV initiations) over the past year. Although the ultimate goal is to reduce accidental needlesticks to zero, the organization might begin with an initial goal to reduce accidental needlesticks during IV initiations to less than 2% in the next 6 months. Because this is a broad objective, additional indicators must be identified to measure the attainment of this objective and analyze the cause.

Performance Indicators

Performance indicators are the actions that measure the attainment of the objective. They must also be specific, attainable, and realistic. Using the objective of reducing needlesticks, some performance indicators might include

- Does not recap needles.
- Disposes of needles in a sharps container with the needle down immediately after use.

As stated above, objectives must be timely. Taking this example one step further, based on technological advancements, the organization might implement a needleless system for IV administration. In order to evaluate the effectiveness of the new system, new performance indicator(s) will need to be developed. One performance indicator might be: Uses a needless system for IV initiation/administration.

Compliance

Compliance with objective/performance indicators involves using available sources of data and information to measure how often personnel comply with the performance indicator. In our example, the compliance level for the objective of decreasing accidental needlesticks during IV initiation is less than 2 percent. In order to determine effectiveness, performance indicators are normally written with the expected compliance level identified. Going back to the original examples:

- Does not recap needles *100 percent of the time*.
- Disposes of needles in a sharps container with the needle down immediately after use *98 percent of the time*.
- Uses a needleless system for IV initiation/administration *100 percent of the time*.

Careful consideration must be given to setting compliance levels. Since the analysis of compliance levels is used to determine the extent to which the objectives have been met, if all objective compliance levels are set at 100 percent, effectiveness of the program is doomed to failure.

There are two primary methods for determining appropriate compliance levels. The first is **benchmarking**. Benchmarking uses comparisons based on data from other organizations, States, or regions. Benchmarking, in some instances, uses national standards. This includes OSHA regulations, NFPA standards, and State law. For example, using personal protective equipment (PPE) and following body substance isolation techniques 100 percent of the time when there is potential exposure to any body fluid is a national standard. This may be another objective of the organization's infection control program. Again this is broad, so performance indicators should be developed that address situations requiring just gloves, situations requiring personal respiratory protection, situations requiring protective eyewear, etc. When there is no standard or accepted compliance level for an objective/performance indicator, the organization must determine the compliance level through data collection and analysis.

INFORMATION MANAGEMENT

When compliance of performance indicator(s) is not met, an analysis must be completed to determine the cause of the problem. Relevant data must be available to complete this analysis. The efficient collection and management of data and their transformation into useful information are fundamental to successful **quality monitoring**. Local, State, and Federal agencies all have specific requirements and/or guidelines that must be included in the infection control program. Therefore, each department will have individual forms and checklists to record the required data.

Data collection also plays a critical role in **program evaluation**. Baseline data collected before implementing a change to the existing program can be compared to later data collected at established intervals. This will provide a clear picture of the progress in attaining program objectives. The data also can be used to identify training needs.

Finally, data collection permits effective **program management** on a day-to-day basis by facilitating various administrative requirements. These include equipment/supplies inventory management, expenditure monitoring, maintenance of employee records, incident analysis, establishing training schedules, etc.

Selection of Data Elements

The elements of data collected should meet the needs of those who will use the information. The data elements must be linked to the program objectives/performance indicators. Determining what data need to be collected should be part of the planning process as program objectives are developed, reviewed, and revised. This may involve modifying existing data elements. Data and information also must be standardized, reliable, rapidly accessible, and timely.

Data should be **standardized**. This means that data sets (what is collected), data definitions, codes, classifications, and terminology are uniform across departments as well as compatible with external databases.

Reliability refers to data being entered consistently. For example, the element of "appropriate protective eye wear worn," could be interpreted as only face shields by some, while others include safety glasses. Reliability hinges on standard definitions of the data elements, and is affected by the motivation of the data collector and the integrity of the storage of the data. Data collection should be automated whenever possible and integrated into work processes. There should be ongoing assessment of data quality. In addition, all those involved in collecting and entering data should be trained so they are knowledgeable about the data being collected and understand how the data are used and the benefits to the organization.

The data also must be **timely** and **rapidly accessible**. Data collection systems vary from simple paper-based records to complex multicomputer systems. For data to be timely and rapidly accessible, the organization must computerize the information collected by other means and integrate other computer data into a central database. This means the organization must have a person whose primary functions are to keep data up-to-date and accurate, conduct analyses, and submit data to State/regional databases.

Regardless of how relevant the data elements are, performance cannot be measured if the analysis program cannot retrieve the needed information. Many commercial software databases are available, but organizations must work with vendors to customize the software to meet their needs. Software also may be developed at the organizational level, if the computer expertise is present.

Types of Infection Control Data

The specific types of data maintained will vary from jurisdiction to jurisdiction, depending on applicable laws, standards, and organizational needs. The following are the most common types of infection control data maintained by emergency response services.

Training

Infection control training (initial and refresher) is necessary to ensure the protection of each emergency responder. Documentation of training reduces potential departmental liability and may be a legal requirement. Training records should document

- Date(s) of the training session
- Subjects covered
- Name(s) and qualifications of instructor(s)
- Names and titles of all individuals attending
- Duration of training
- Test scores or other indications of satisfactory performance

It is helpful if the information system also includes the responders' certifications and the expiration dates of those certifications so qualifications can be tracked and training records can be compared with established training requirements. In this way, individual training needs can be identified, and organizational trends and priorities can be analyzed. OSHA requires that training records on infection control be maintained for 3 years from the date the training occurred.

Exposures

All exposures to communicable disease must be documented. Exposure documentation ensures compliance with jurisdictional regulations and protection of members and their families. It also can be used to identify trends that may indicate the need for new training requirements and/or modification of existing protocols. Exposure records should include

- Date of incident
- Location of incident
- Incident number

- Route of exposure

- PPE used

- Type of exposure, if known

- Member's name

- Description of member's duties as they relate to this exposure

- Social Security Number (required by OSHA)

- Description of incident and circumstances under which the exposure occurred

- Notifications made

- Treatment and follow-up provided

Figure 5-2 is an example of an exposure form.

Figure 5-2

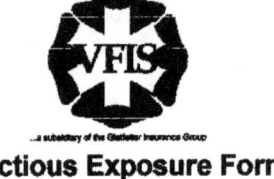

...a subsidiary of the Glatfelter Insurance Group

Infectious Exposure Form

Exposed Member's Name: _____ Position: _____

Soc. Sec. #: _____ Home Phone: _____

Field Inc. #: _____ Shift: _____ Company: _____

Name of Patient: _____ Sex: _____

Age: _____ Address: _____

Suspected or Confirmed Disease: _____

Transported to: _____

Transported by: _____

Date of Exposure: _____ Time of Exposure: _____

Type of Incident (auto accident, trauma): _____

Type of protective equipment utilized: _____

What where you exposed to:

Blood _____ Tears _____ Feces _____ Urine _____ Saliva _____

Vomitus _____ Sputum _____ Sweat _____ Other _____

What part(s) of your body became exposed? Be specific: _____

_____

_____

_____

_____

Did you have any open cuts, sores, or rashes that became exposed? Be specific: _____

_____

_____

How did exposure occur? Be specific: _____

_____

_____

Did you seek medical attention? _____Yes _____No

Where? _____ Date: _____

Contact Infection Control Supervisor: Date_____ Time: _____

Supervisor's Signature: _____ Date: _____

Member's Signature: _____ Date: _____

It is important to remember that all exposure records are **confidential**. It will be necessary to establish passwords in computerized systems to prevent unauthorized access to records. Analytical report formats should not include individual names or other identifying information unless necessary. Similarly, information from the system should not be distributed to persons without a need to know.

OSHA requires exposure records be retained for the duration of employment plus 30 years. This may require transfer of the records to a separate system: Microfilm may be used. It also should be considered that the programs currently being used to store exposure records will be outdated in 30 years, so original records may not be retrievable.

Personal Health Data

The department must establish and maintain an accurate personal medical health record for each member. The medical record should be up-to-date and include

- Name of member
- Results of all medical examinations (pre-entry, pre-assignment, annual/ongoing, and post-exposure)
- Medical diagnoses and recommendations
- Treatment and prescriptions
- Immunization record, including hepatitis B
- Follow-up procedures and post-exposure evaluations
- Member medical complaints and symptoms
- Record of medically caused work restrictions

Like exposure records, medical records are confidential, and can be released only to authorized individuals with the written consent of the member. Medical records should not be kept with other personnel records. Protection of member/employee medical records and the requirement that medical records be retained for the duration of employment plus 30 years is covered in 29 CFR Part 1910.20.

Work Practices

The department must record data on work practices at the scene and in the station to be able to evaluate whether safety is being maintained. Collection of these data will fulfill applicable legal compliance and quality monitoring requirements. Regular observation of employee behavior at emergency incidents and in the station is necessary to evaluate compliance with established protocols and work practices. Areas that require monitoring include

- Compliance with infection control protocols (i.e., appropriate use of PPE)
- Storage facilities (conspicuously marked and secured)
- Disinfecting areas (marked, contaminants isolated)
- Disposal areas (marked, containers secured, waste disposal logs up-to-date)
- Compliance with applicable laws/regulations

Compliance monitoring can be accomplished by using specific audit forms based on jurisdictional requirements. Analysis results should be documented and maintained. All deficiencies noted should include recommendations for improvement and follow-up re-inspections.

Equipment and Supplies Inventory

All infection control equipment and supplies must be available. This can be accomplished only through an accurate and efficient inventory system. The inventory list must identify all items necessary for the program. For each item, the inventory should document

- Cost
- Minimum on-hand requirement
- Expiration date
- Current stock balance
- Date/Amount ordered
- Date received
- Date/Amount issued
- Organization/Individual receiving the supplies

Additional Data Types

Several additional types of data may contribute to information regarding the effectiveness of the infection control program. **Employee interviews** can be used to determine individual knowledge and acceptance of infection control protocols. Post-incident analyses or individual debriefing after an emergency response can also help identify areas of confusion that can be addressed in counseling and/or training sessions.

Incident run sheets can help identify unexpected trends within the system. For example, an increase in response volume will require increased supplies and equipment. This affects inventory supply and the need to re-order. It may also require increases in future budget requests.

Monitoring **compensation claims** will help identify trends in injuries and exposures. Analysis of these claims can provide direction for possible training, behavior modification needs, and/or protocol changes.

The department also should monitor **community health trends** to stay current on prevalent communicable diseases, potentially dangerous situations, etc. Monitoring community trends facilitates a proactive infection control response to unexpected threats. For example, if there is an outbreak of meningitis within the community, the department could take immediate early action to notify all members and implement more stringent infection control procedures.

Confidentiality

Maintaining the confidentiality of certain records is necessary for the protection of both employees and patients. Each individual's right to privacy is guaranteed by law and each State/municipality has enacted "privacy laws" that regulate information release and record retention.

All **patient-related information** is confidential. Each department should have standard operating procedures (SOP's) covering the release of patient information, since inadvertent release of confidential information can result in civil liability. Patient information should be released only to authorized individuals, and in accordance with current guidelines and regulations regarding patient privacy, need for consent, and (if a research study) approval of appropriate supervisory bodies. All inquiries and the release of patient information should be documented and stored. The records should include a copy of the authorization for release, the name of the individual receiving the information, the name of the individual releasing the information, and the dates involved.

Members' medical records also are confidential. While exposure records may be used to evaluate the effectiveness of the program, the confidentiality of the members involved must be maintained. The types and numbers of exposures can be audited, but names must not be used. Written procedures should specify who has access to medical records and under what circumstances. The process by which medical information is collected, stored, retrieved, and released must be thought out carefully. Release of medical information should occur only with the written consent of the member. The consent form should include

- Date of written authorization
- Name and signature of member authorizing release of information
- Name of individual authorized to receive medical information
- Description of medical information to be released
- General description of the purpose for release of medical information
- Date the written authorization expires

It is critical that members' medical records are not disclosed or reported to any person within or outside the department except as required by law. The original medical records should stay in the department medical file. Only copies of this information should be released with proper authorization.

Computer security must be designed to protect the confidentiality of patient and member medical records. This may require the use of passwords to limit access to a minimum of individuals. Logs should be maintained to document the release of information. Access to the computer or computer terminals must be secured. (This also applies to written records in a filing system.) Only authorized personnel should have access to the password or secure areas that contain medical records. The issuance of authorization, keys, etc., should be recorded and monitored. The department should take full advantage of legal resources available for guidance on statutory requirements related to confidentiality.

PROGRAM REVISION

Program revision occurs as the result of three primary causes. Changes in laws/regulations or technology may require revisions in protocols or equipment related to infection control. Program revision may also be necessary when information analysis reveals lack of compliance of performance indicators.

Laws/Regulations

As stated earlier in this manual, it is critical that the infection control officer stay current on the laws/regulations governing infection control practices. Reviewing *Morbidity Mortality Weekly* on a regular basis is an excellent resource for finding changes in suggested practices and updating knowledge of infectious/communicable diseases. Establishing a relationship with local infection control specialists in hospitals is also a resource that should be helpful in maintaining up-to-date information.

Non-compliance

When compliance set for a performance indicator is not met, an analysis must be completed to determine the cause of the problem. For example, an infection control performance objective is that personnel will use body substance isolation techniques 100 percent of the time when there is potential exposure to any body fluid. Compliance is determined to be only 85 percent. A careful analysis might identify one or more of the following reasons for the non-compliance, each of which may require action steps at different levels of the system.

Possible reason: Personnel are not following protocol.

    a.   Personnel are not familiar with specific infection control protocols.

    b.   Personnel do not know which situations require specific PPE (e.g., eyewear during intubation)

    c.   PPE interferes, or is perceived to interfere with task performance.

Possible reason: Inadequate supplies of PPE.

    a.   Increased call volume depleted supplies.

    b.   There is a distribution problem

    c.   There is a supplier problem.

Possible reason: Personnel respond directly to the scene without adequate PPE.

    a.   Protocols are inadequate or unclear.

    b.   There is an inadequate supply of PPE.

    c.   Personnel do not maintain appropriate PPE in personal vehicles.

From this limited example, it is obvious that analyzing causes of non-compliance involves the entire organization and system, including policymakers, line personnel, health and safety personnel, and others.

ACTION PLAN

Developing the Plan

Once the analysis is completed, an action plan needs to be developed to correct the cause(s) of the problem. The action plan should be specific, with exact steps necessary to assure compliance. The first decision that management must make is who will be on the team that develops the action plan. In addition to the infection control officer, the team should include representatives directly affected by the performance indicator, including line personnel. A timeframe for both the completion of the action plan and the accomplishment of the actions should be identified. Providing the team with a schedule and checkpoints for completion of the plan helps keep them on-task to reach a solution in an acceptable timeframe.

In addition to identifying the specific steps necessary to correct the problem, two additional areas should be addressed when developing the action plan. First, obstacles that might impede the implementation of the plan should be identified. Examples of obstacles include lack of resources or lack of funding. Second, resources needed to carry out the plan should be identified. These resources might include equipment, funding, and/or training programs.

Implementing the Plan

In addition to the obvious necessity of allocating resources, the biggest challenge during project implementation will be to maintain credibility and focus, and to maintain momentum among team members.

- **Follow the schedule** -- This may seem rather obvious, but often it is not done. Efficient use of the schedule will help concentrate efforts and attention where they are most needed. It also will help anticipate the next steps. Schedules enhance coordination and communication within a team. Everyone should be able to identify where they are at any given point, and know others' responsibilities.

- **Empower team members** -- Provide the resources and authority to accomplish the task, and **allow** the team members to do what they do best.

- <u>**Keep others informed**</u> -- This is an obvious component, but one that is often neglected or ignored during critical periods. Schedule communication opportunities, and carry through.

Monitor the Plan

Once the plan is implemented, it is critical that the results of the implementation be monitored and evaluated to determine results or problems that arise. Monitoring and evaluation may take a variety of forms, depending on the actions specified in the plan. Methods to collect data to monitor results should be developed during the planning stage. It is important that the monitoring methods allow for timely feedback, so any problems will be detected early. If problems with the plan are detected during the monitoring phase, or if the action plan did not make a difference, it must be revised. Based on the problem identified, revision may require re-entering the process cycle at any point.

SUMMARY

Infection control principles and practices are being updated constantly. Therefore, the department's infection control program must be evaluated regularly and revised to ensure continuing effectiveness. Periodic evaluations ensure continued compliance with current standards and practices.

Infection control data collection and analysis are critical for effective program evaluation, compliance/quality monitoring, and ongoing program management. Detailed records must be maintained in the areas of training, exposure, incidents, health, work practices, and equipment/supplies inventories. The confidentiality of patient-related information and members' medical/exposure records must be assured. The department should seek a legal review of all program changes prior to implementation, since infection control programs deal with medical and legal issues and member safety.

SECTION 6

SPECIAL SITUATIONS

OVERVIEW

This chapter will cover infection control considerations for two special situations: the training environment and practices for protecting the patient.

THE TRAINING ENVIRONMENT

Two aspects of training are addressed: training in context and the cleaning and disinfecting of equipment.

Training in Context

For many years training has reinforced the use of personal protective equipment (PPE) when dealing with the potential for exposure to blood or body fluids. There are few services left where providers do not don protective gloves when dealing with patients. However, the same cannot be said about the use of eyewear, masks, and gowns.

Training programs should consistently stress the use of **appropriate** PPE in lectures and discussions. Training programs also should reinforce using the appropriate PPE needed in "hands on" practice stations. Testing stations for the National Registry Examination (both basic and advanced levels) require the provider to use body substance isolation (BSI). Although this concept usually is reinforced verbally, frequently it is accepted as being met when the student demonstrates the donning of gloves only.

It is a well-known educational fact that the way we learn a process/skill in the training environment is the way we tend to carry that process out in real life. A second educational fact is that it is very difficult to change the steps of a work process/skill from the way it was initially learned. When the training environment allows students to don only gloves as a demonstration of the use of PPE, this practice frequently is carried into the real world of patient care.

Training programs can increase compliance with the use of appropriate BSI by developing a variety of "hands on" scenarios that require providers to don PPE in addition to gloves. Such scenarios might include an airway management case that requires protective eyewear and a mask, or the assessment of a potential tuberculosis patient that requires the use of respiratory protection that meets Occupational Safety and Health Administration (OSHA) standards. If providers practice skills using **all** the PPE dictated by the situation, they are far more likely to use all the equipment in the job environment.

Those responsible for planning and conducting training should assess the need for training in context, provide supplies of PPE adequate to allow all attendees to complete the training exercises using the appropriate PPE, and notify attendees to bring any personally fitted PPE needed with them to training sessions.

Cleaning Equipment

Risk of disease transmission using manikins is extremely low. According to the American Heart Association, as of March 2000 there were no reports of infection associated with direct contact with manikins during CPR training.[6]

Since there is some risk of disease transmission, manikin surfaces should be cleaned and disinfected after each use. Cleaning means washing the equipment with soap and water. Disinfecting involves the use of a disinfectant to kill many of the microorganisms that may be on the object. There are many types of manikins, so cleaning and disinfecting should follow the specific manufacturer's guidelines. Internal parts such as artificial lungs and valve mechanisms should be cleaned thoroughly between users.

The human immunodeficiency virus (HIV) is inactivated in less than 10 minutes at room temperature by a number of commercial disinfectants. An equally effective and less expensive alternative to commercial disinfectants is a bleach solution. One part bleach to 100 parts water (1:100, approximately 2 cups/gallon) should be effective for training equipment, as long as the equipment is first washed with warm, soapy water and

---

[6] American Heart Association. (2000). Guidelines for cardiopulmonary resuscitation and emergency cardiovascular care; Supplement to *Circulation*; 12(8).

rinsed with clean water. Follow manufacturers' instructions for commercial disinfectants.

PROTECTING THE PATIENT

Guidelines for job functions for health-care workers infected with HIV or Hepatitis B virus (HBV) are addressed in *Recommendations for Preventing Transmission of Human Immunodeficiency Virus and Hepatitis B Virus to Patients During Exposure-Prone Invasive Procedures* (MMWR Vol. 40, No. RR-08, July 12, 1991) and *Guidelines for the Management of Occupational Exposures to HBV, HCV and HIV and Recommendations for Postexposure Prophylaxis* (MMWR, May 15, 2001). These recommendations are summarized in Chapter 2 of this Guide. The major focus of infected workers providing care revolves around invasive procedures that might result in exposing the patient to the virus. Although the recommendations are made for hospital workers, intravenous initiation often occurs in confined spaces or under conditions of poor visibility in the out-of-hospital area. Therefore, this is a legitimate concern in emergency services.

The work status of an infected worker also may be a legal issue under the Americans with Disability Act (ADA). Some contagious diseases, including HIV infection and tuberculosis (TB), are considered disabilities under the ADA. Relieving an "otherwise qualified" employee with a communicable disease must be supported by objective evidence of risk, and reasonable accommodation to eliminate that risk must have been attempted.

Health-care workers who are infected with HIV or HBV should receive counseling from an expert review panel, including the department physician and the employee's personal physician and receive advice regarding under what circumstances, if any, they may perform invasive procedures. If these workers are allowed to continue to perform invasive procedures, there may be an obligation to notify patients of their positive HIV/HBV status before the procedure is initiated.

If counseling results in the prohibition of invasive procedures, the worker should be provided opportunities to continue appropriate patient care activities whenever possible. If the worker is removed from patient care due to strong risk, career counseling and job retraining should be available to allow continued employment in another appropriate area. If the worker's practices are modified because of HBV infection, he/she should be reevaluated periodically to determine whether the seropositive status changes due to resolution of infection or as a result of treatment

SUMMARY

The training environment and the infected worker are two special situations that must be considered in the department's overall infection control program. Infection control practices in the training environment should reflect the infection control practices required in the field. To reinforce appropriate infection control practices, training programs should develop a variety of scenarios that require the use of all PPE. Practicing with appropriate PPE will increase the compliance of using that equipment when needed in the actual job environment. Although there has been no documented transmission of infection from manikins, training programs must remain vigilant in cleaning and disinfecting the equipment used in an educational setting by following the manufacturer's suggested guidelines.

Workers with HIV and tuberculosis are protected under ADA. The scope of practice for workers with HIV and HBV relative to invasive procedures is addressed in the Center for Disease Control and Prevention's (CDC) *Recommendations for Preventing Transmission of Human Immunodeficiency Virus and Hepatitis B Virus to Patients During Exposure-Prone Invasive Procedures* and *Guidelines for the Management of Occupational Exposures to HBV, HCV and HIV and Recommendations for Postexposure Prophylaxis* (MMWR, May 15, 2001). Restricting the scope of practice of an infected worker should be preceded by counsel from an expert panel that includes the fire department physician and the member's personal physician. If practice is restricted, the worker should be allowed to continue appropriate patient care activities whenever possible or provided job retraining to allow continued employment in another appropriate area. If the worker is HBV positive, he/she should be reevaluated periodically to determine whether the positive status changes due to resolution of infection or as a result of treatment

BIBLIOGRAPHY

BIBLIOGRAPHY

Barillo, D. (1997). Infection control In Pons, P. & Cason, D. (Eds.). *Paramedic Field Care* (131-144). American College of Emergency Physicians St. Louis: Mosby YearBook.

Bolyard, E.A., Tablan, O.C., Williams W.W., Pearson, M., Shapiro, C.N., Deitchman, S.D. & Hospital Infection Control Practices Advisory Committee. (1998). Guidelines for infection control in health care personnel. *American Journal of Infection Control* 26; 289-354 and *Infection Control and Hospital Epidemiology* 19; 407-463.

Dickinson E. (1999). Infection control and body substance isolation. *Fire Service Emergency Care* (35-50). Upper Saddle River, NJ: Prentice-Hall, Inc.

Mistovich J., Hafen, B., & Karren, K. (2000) Ambulance operations. *Prehospital Emergency Care* (810-830). Upper Saddle River, NJ: Prentice-Hall, Inc.

National Fire Academy. (1999). Student Manual*: Advanced leadership issues in EMS.* Emmitsburg, MD: NFA.

_____. (1992). Student Manual*: Infection control for emergency response personnel: The supervisor's role*. Emmitsburg, MD: NFA.

_____. (1998). Student Manual*: Management of emergency medical services.* Emmitsburg, MD: NFA.

National Fire Protection Association. (1997). NFPA 1500: *Standard on fire department occupational safety and health program*. Quincy, MA: NFPA.

_____. (1997b). NFPA 1521: *Standard on fire department safety officer*. Quincy, MA: NFPA.

_____. (2000). NFPA 1581: *Standard on fire department infection control program.* Quincy, MA: NFPA.

_____. (2000b). NFPA 1582: *Standard on medical requirements for fire fighters and information for fire department physicians*. Quincy, MA: NFPA.

National Highway and Transportation Safety Administration. (1997). *A leadership guide to quality improvement for emergency medical services (EMS) systems.*

U.S. Department of Health and Human Services, Centers for Disease Control. (1994). Guidelines for preventing the transmission of mycobacterium tuberculosis in health-care facilities. *Morbidity Mortality Weekly Report*. Vol. 43, No. RR-13.

_____. (1989). Guidelines for prevention of transmission of human immunodeficiency virus and hepatitis B Virus to health care and public safety workers. *Morbidity Mortality Weekly Report.* Vol. 38, No.2-6.

_____. (1997). Immunization of health-care workers: Recommendations of the advisory committee on immunization practices (ACIP) and the hospital infection control practices advisory committee (HICPAC). *Morbidity Mortality Weekly Report.* Vol. 46, No. RR-18.

_____. (1998). Public health service guidelines for the management of health-care worker exposures to HIV and recommendations for post exposure prophylaxis. *Morbidity Mortality Weekly Report.* Vol. 47, No. RR-7.

_____. (1991). Recommendations for preventing transmission of human immunodeficiency virus and hepatitis B virus to patients during exposure-prone invasive procedures. *Morbidity Mortality Weekly Report.* Vol. 40, No. RR-08.

_____. (1998). Recommendations for prevention and control of hepatitis C virus (HCV) infection and HCV-related chronic disease. *Morbidity Mortality Weekly Report.* Vol. 47, No. 19.

_____. (1999). *Preventing occupational HIV transmission to health care workers.*

_____. (2000). Recommendations for prevention and control of mennigococcal disease. *Morbidity Mortality Weekly Report.* Vol. 49, No. RR-07.

_____. (1987). Recommendations for prevention of HIV transmission in health-care settings. *Morbidity Mortality Weekly Report.* Vol. 36 No.2

_____. (2000b). Updated U.S. Public Health Service guidelines for the management for occupational exposures to HBV, HCV, and HIV and recommendations for postexposure prophylaxis. *Morbidity Mortality Weekly Report.* Vol. 50, No. 11.

_____. (1988). Universal precautions for prevention of transmission of human immunodeficiency virus, hepatitis B virus, and other bloodborne pathogens in health care settings. *Morbidity Mortality Weekly Report.* Vol. 37, No. 24.

_____. National Center for HIV, STD, and TB Prevention. *Reported tuberculosis in the United States, 1999.* http://www.cdc.gov/nchstp/tb/surv/surv99/surv99.htm.

_____. (1999). National Institute for Occupational Safety and Health. *Preventing needlestick injuries in health care settings,* Pub. No.2000-108.

U.S. Department of Labor, Occupational Safety and Health Administration. (1991). *Occupational exposure to bloodborne pathogens: Final rule (29 CFR Part 1910.1030).* Washington, DC: Federal Register. Vol. 56, No. 235.

_____. (1997). *Safer needle devices: Protecting health care workers.* Washington, DC.

_____. (1999). *Enforcement procedures for the occupational exposure to bloodborne pathogens (CPL 2-2.44D).* Washington, DC.

U.S. Environmental Protection Agency, Office of Solid Waste. (1986). *EPA guide for infectious waste management.* Washington, DC.

U.S. Fire Administration. (1999). *Developing effective standard operating procedures for fire and EMS departments.* Federal Emergency Management Agency: Washington, D.C.

_____. (1992). *Guide to developing and managing an emergency service infection control program.* Federal Emergency Management Agency: Washington, DC.

_____. (1997). *Safety and health considerations for the design of fire and emergency medical services stations.* Federal Emergency Management Agency: Washington, DC.

APPENDICES

A. Glossary of Common Terms
B. Laws, Standards, and Guidelines
C. Sources of Additional Information

APPENDIX A

GLOSSARY OF COMMON TERMS

GLOSSARY OF COMMON TERMS

AIDS: Acquired Immune Deficiency Syndrome, a communicable disease caused by Human Immunodeficiency Virus (HIV).

Advanced Life Support (ALS): Emergency medical treatment at an advanced level, usually provided by paramedics, and including use of drugs, cardiac monitoring and intervention, and intravenous fluids.

Airborne Pathogen: Pathologic microorganisms spread by droplets expelled into the air or aerosol, typically through a productive cough or sneeze.

Antibody: A component of the immune system which eliminates or counteracts a foreign substance (antigen) in the body.

Antigen: A foreign substance which stimulates the production of antibodies in the immune system.

ARC (AIDS-Related Complex): An outdated term used to describe symptoms of HIV infection in patients who have not developed AIDS. These include fatigue, diarrhea, night sweats, and enlarged lymph nodes. ARC is not included in the current CDC classification of HIV infection.

Bacteria: A type of living microorganism that can produce disease in a suitable host. Bacteria can self-reproduce, and some forms may produce toxins harmful to their host.

Basic Life Support (BLS): "Emergency medical treatment at a level authorized to be performed by emergency medical technicians as defined by the medical authority having jurisdiction" (NFPA 1500). Generally refers to treatment provided at EMT-B levels.

Biohazard: A risk of exposure to harmful bacteria, viruses, or other dangerous biological agents

Bloodborne Pathogen: Pathologic microorganisms that are present in human blood and that can cause disease in humans. (OSHA) Note: the term "blood" includes blood, blood components, and products made from human blood.

Body Fluids: "Fluids that have been recognized by the CDC as directly linked to the transmission of HIV and/or HBV and/or to which Universal Precautions apply: blood, semen, blood products, vaginal secretions, cerebrospinal fluid, synovial fluid, pericardial fluid, amniotic fluid, and concentrated HIV or HBV viruses." (OSHA)

Body Substance Isolation (BSI): An infection control strategy that considers all body substances potentially infectious. This protective measure is accomplished through barrier protection using personal protective equipment (gloves, masks, protective eyewear, gowns, and resuscitation devices, as appropriate) to prevent personal contact with any body fluids or other potentially infectious material.

CDC (Centers for Disease Control and Prevention): A branch of the Department of Health and Human Services, Public Health Service, that serves as the national focus for developing and applying disease prevention and control, environmental health, and health promotion and education activities designed to improve the health of the people of the United States.

Chickenpox (Varicella): A vaccine-preventable, highly communicable disease caused by a herpes virus resulting in skin vesicles. Commonly occurs in childhood.

CISD (Critical Incident Stress Debriefing): Stress reduction processes designed to address the special needs of emergency response personnel in dealing with situations which cause strong emotional reactions or interfere with the ability to function.

Cleaning: The physical removal of dirt and debris, generally accomplished with soap and water and physical scrubbing. (NFPA 1581)

Communicable (Contagious) Disease: A disease that can be transmitted from one person to another.

Contamination: Soiling or pollution, as by the introduction of organisms into a wound or onto equipment.

Debilitating Illness or Injury: "A condition that temporarily or permanently prevents a member of the fire department from engaging in normal duties and activities as a result of illness or injury." (NFPA 1500)

Decontamination: The use of physical or chemical means to remove, inactivate, or destroy bloodborne, airborne, or foodborne pathogens on a surface or item to the point they are not longer capable of transmitting infectious particles. (NFPA 1581)

Disease: An alteration of health, with a characteristic set of symptoms, which may affect the entire body or specific organs.

> **Contagious:** Infectious disease that can be transmitted from one person to another from either direct or indirect contact.

> **Infectious:** Disease due to a pathogenic microorganism such as a bacteria, virus, or fungus.

Disease Transmission:

> **Direct:** Communicable disease is transmitted from one person to another due to direct contact with infected blood, body fluids, or other infectious material.

> **Indirect:** Communicable disease is transmitted from one person to another without direct contact.

> **Infectious:** An illness or disease resulting from invasion of a host by disease-producing organisms such as bacteria, viruses, fungi, or parasites.

Disinfection: "A procedure which inactivates virtually all recognized pathogenic microorganisms, but not necessarily all microbial forms (ex. Bacterial endospores) or inanimate objects." (OSHA)

ELISA: Enzyme-linked immunosorbent assay. A test used to detect antibodies to the AIDS virus, indicating infection. For accuracy, a positive ELISA test is always repeated. If still positive, a Western Blot test is then performed to confirm the diagnosis.

Emergency Medical Care: The provision of treatment to patients, including first aid, cardiopulmonary resuscitation, basic life support, advanced life support a, and other medical procedures that occur prior to arrival at a hospital or other health-care facility. (NFPA 1581)

Emergency Medical Operations: Delivery of emergency medical care and transportation prior to arrival at a hospital or other health care facility. (NFPA 1581)

EMS (Emergency Medical Services): A group, department, or agency that is trained and equipped to respond in an organized manner to any emergency situation where there is the potential need for the delivery of prehospital emergency medical care and/or transportation. EMS can be provided by fire department, private, third service, or hospital-based systems or any combination thereof.

Enteric Precautions: A system of precautions to prevent transmission of disease by the oral/fecal route.

Etiologic Agent: The agent that is the cause or origin of a disease.

Exposure: Eye, mouth, other mucous membrane, non-related skin, or parenteral contact with blood, other body fluids, or other potentially infectious material.

> **Parenteral:** "Exposure which occurs through a break in the skin barrier." (OSHA) Includes injections, needle sticks, human bites, and cuts contaminated with blood.

First Responder: Personnel who arrive first on the scene at emergency incidents and have the responsibility to act. Includes fire, police, EMS, and other public safety workers.

Fluid Resistant Clothing: Clothing designed and constructed to provide a barrier against accidental contact with body fluids.

Fungus: A group of microorganisms including molds and yeasts, similar to the cellular structure of plants. Some fungi can cause disease.

German Measles: See Rubella.

Gloves, Emergency Medical: Single-use, patient examination gloves that are designed to provide a barrier against body fluids meeting. (NFPA 1581)

Gonorrhea: A sexually transmitted disease caused by the bacteria *Neisseria gonorrhea.*

Health-Care Worker: "An employee of a health care facility including, but not limited to, nurses, physicians, dentists, and other dental workers, optometrists, podiatrists, chiropractors, laboratory and blood bank technologists and technician, research laboratory scientists, phlebotomists, dialysis personnel, **paramedics, emergency medical technicians,** medical examiners, morticians, housekeepers, laundry workers, **and others whose work may involve direct contact with body fluids** from living individuals or corpses." (OSHA, bold added.)

Health Database: "A compilation of records and data relating to the health experience of a group of individuals, maintained in such a manner that it is retrievable for study and analysis over a period of time." (NFPA 1581)

Health Promotion: "Preventive health activities that identify real and potential risks in the work environment, and that inform, motivate, and otherwise help people to adopt and maintain healthy practices and lifestyles." (NFPA 1500)

Health and Safety Officer: "The member of the fire department assigned and authorized by the fire chief as the manager of the safety and health program and who performs the duties and responsibilities specified in NFPA 1581." (NFPA 1581)

Hepatitis: Inflammation or swelling of the liver. Hepatitis can be caused by certain drugs, toxins, or infectious agents, including viruses. Hepatitis caused by viruses include A,B, C, D, E, F G, and other, as yet unclassified, types.

> **Hepatitis A (Infectious):** Viral infection normally spread by fecal contamination.

Hepatitis B (HBV, Serum): Viral infection spread through blood contact, and also as a sexually transmitted disease. Infection may result in chronic hepatitis, liver cancer, cirrhosis of the liver, or death.

Hepatitis C (HCV): Viral infection spread through blood contact. Currently, no prophylaxis is available.

Hepatitis D (HDV, Delta): Viral infection occurring in people with present or past HBV infection. A complication of HBV infection and can increase the severity of HBV infection.

Hepatitis E: Viral infection spread by the fecal-oral route.

Hepatitis F: Viral infection with mode of transmission unknown, but may be bloodborne.

Hepatitis G: Viral infection spread through blood contact.

Herpes: A family of similar viruses which can cause different diseases, including chickenpox, zoster, "cold sores," and genital herpes type II.

Zoster (Shingles): A painful skin rash caused by recurrence of a past case of chickenpox. Herpes zoster is not typically spread person-to-person, but persons who have not had chickenpox previously can contract chickenpox after exposure to a patient with zoster.

HIV Infection (HIV Positive): A person who has tested positive for HIV antibodies on two ELISA tests, confirmed with Western Blot testing. HIV-infected patients can spread the virus through blood and body fluids.

Host: The person who harbors or nourishes a disease-producing organism.

Human Immunodeficiency Virus: The causative agent of AIDS. HIV type 1 causes most cases of AIDS. A second virus, HIV-2 is a less common cause of the disease.

Iatrogenic: A complication, injury, or disease state resulting from medical treatment.

Immediately Dangerous to Life or Health (IDLH): "Any atmosphere that poses an immediate hazard to life or produces immediate irreversible debilitating effects on health." (NFPA 1500).

Immunization: The process of rendering a person immune, or highly resistant to a disease.

Incident Commander: "The person in overall command of an emergency incident." (NFPA 1500)

Incident Management System (IMS): "An organized system of roles, responsibilities, and standard operating procedures used to manage emergency operations" (NFPA 1500) Such system often is referred to as an Incident Command System.

Incubation Period: The time from exposure to the disease until the first appearance of symptoms.

Infection: Growth of pathogenic organisms in the tissues of a host, with or without detectable signs of injury.

Infection Control Officer: "The person within the fire department who is responsible for managing the department infection control program and for coordinating efforts surrounding the investigation of an exposure." (NFPA 1581)

Infection Control Practitioner: A medical professional with a specialty interest in infection control.

Infection Control Program: "The establishment's oral or written policy and implementation of procedures relating to the control of infectious disease hazards where employees may be exposed to direct contact with body fluids." (OSHA)

Infectious: Capable of causing infection in a suitable host.

Infectious Waste: "Blood and blood products, pathological wastes, microbiological wastes, and contaminated sharps." (MMWR)

Joint Advisory Notice: A list of recommendations developed by the Department of Labor/Department of Health and Human Services to assist employers in implementing the Centers for Disease Control and Prevention guidelines.

Leakproof Bag: A bag that is sufficiently sturdy to prevent tearing or breaking and can be sealed securely to prevent leakage. Such bags are red in color or display the universal biohazard symbol. (NFPA 1581)

Measles: A vaccine-preventable viral communicable disease causing a skin rash. Usually occurs in childhood.

Member: "A person involved in performing the duties and responsibilities of a fire department, under the auspices of the organization. A member can be full-time, part-time, paid, or unpaid, can occupy any position or rank within the fire department, and might or might not engage in emergency operations." (NFPA 1581)

Member Assistance Program: "A generic term used to describe the various methods used in the workplace for the control of alcohol and other substance abuse, stress, and personal problems that adversely affect job performance." (NFPA 1500)

Meningitis: An infection of the meninges (layers covering the brain and spinal cord). May be caused by a bacteria or virus; considered a communicable disease.

Microorganism: A living organism, usually visible only with a microscope, including bacteria, viruses, fungi, and parasites.

Morbidity and Mortality Weekly Report (MMWR): A weekly publication from the Centers for Disease Control and Prevention presenting up-to-date information on communicable diseases.

Mucous Membrane: The lining of the nose, mouth, eyes, vagina, and rectum. Mucous membranes are not as durable as other skin; contact of infected body fluids with intact mucous membranes may transmit disease.

Mumps: A vaccine-preventable virus resulting in inflamed and swollen parotid glands. Usually occurring in childhood.

Nosocomial: Originating in the hospital.

Occupational: Related to the performance of duties and responsibilities of the job.

> **Exposure:** "Reasonably anticipated skin, eye, mucous membrane, or parenteral contact with blood or other potentially infectious materials that may result from the performance of an employee's duties." (OSHA) This definition excludes incidental exposures that may take place on the job, that are neither reasonable or routinely expected, and that the worker is not required to incur in the normal course of employment.

> **Illness:** "An illness or disease contracted through or aggravated by the performance of the duties, responsibilities, and functions of a fire department member." (NFPA 1500)

> **Injury:** "An injury sustained during the performance of the duties, responsibilities, and functions of a fire department member." (NFPA 1500).

Pathogen: A microorganism that can cause disease. Pathogens can be bacteria, viruses, fungi, or parasites.

Personal Protective Equipment (PPE): "Specialized clothing or equipment worn by an employee for protection from a hazard. General work clothes (e.g. uniforms, pants, shirts, or blouses) not intended to function as protection against a hazard are not considered to be personal protective equipment." (OSHA)

Phlebotomist: Any health care worker who draws blood samples. (OSHA)

Pneumocyctis Pneumonia: A type of pneumonia caused by a parasite, seen in patients with impaired immune systems.

Purified Protein Derivative (PPD): A skin test for exposure to tuberculosis.

Recombinant Vaccine: A vaccine produced by genetic manipulation (gene splicing), usually in yeast.

RPR: A blood test for syphilis.

Rubella: A vaccine-preventable viral disease. Rubella infection during pregnancy can cause birth defects.

Sexually Transmitted Disease (STD): A disease spread through sexual contact or activities. HIV and HBV are both bloodborne and sexually transmitted diseases.

Seroconversion: A change in the status of one's serum test. For example, someone initially tests negative for HIV, then tests positive at a later date.

Sharps: "Any object that can penetrate the skin including, but not limited to needles, lancets, scalpels, and broken capillary tubes." (OSHA)

Sharps Container: "Container that is closable, puncture-resistant, disposable, and leakproof on the sides and bottom; red in color or displays the universal biohazard symbol; and designed to store sharp objects after use." (NFPA 1581)

Standard Precautions: "Synthesize the major features of universal precautions and body substance isolation and applies them to all patients receiving care in the hospital. Apply to blood, all body fluids except sweat regardless of whether or not they contain visible blood, non-intact skin, and mucous membranes." (CDC)

Sterilization: "The use of a physical or chemical procedure to destroy all microbial life, including highly resistant bacterial endospores." (OSHA)

Syphilis: A sexually transmitted infectious disease. Syphilis is uncommonly transmitted through blood exposure or transfusion.

Tuberculocidal: Capable of killing tuberculosis bacteria. Used as a guideline for effectiveness of disinfecting/sterilizing agents.

Tuberculosis (TB): A communicable disease caused by the bacteria *Mycobacterium tuberculosis*, usually affecting the lungs.

Universal Precautions: Infection control strategy developed by the CDC for **hospital workers**. Universal precautions are based on the concept that blood and **certain** body fluids (any body fluids containing visible blood, semen, vaginal secretions, tissues, cerebrospinal fluid (CSF), synovial fluid, pleural fluid, peritoneal fluid, pericardial fluid, and amniotic fluid) of all patients should be considered potentially infectious for HIV, HBV, and other bloodborne pathogens.

Vaccine: A suspension of attenuated or killed microorganisms (bacteria, viruses or rickettsiae), administered to prevent or reduce the chance of contracting infectious diseases.

VDRL: Blood test for syphilis. Stands for Venereal Disease Research Laboratory, where the test was designed.

Venereal: Due to or propagated by sexual contact.

Virulence: The disease-evoking power of a microorganism in a given host.

Virus: A microorganism usually only visible with the electron microscope. Normally reside within other living (host) cells and cannot reproduce outside a living cell.

Western Blot: A test for HIV, used to confirm a positive ELISA test. More expensive and time consuming that the ELISA, but more specific. Diagnosis of HIV infection requires two positive ELISA tests, confirmed with a positive Western Blot test.

Whitlow: A fingertip infection commonly caused by herpes virus. Spread by contact with respiratory secretions.

Window Phase: The time from exposure to the disease to positive testing.

APPENDIX B

LAWS, REGULATIONS, AND STANDARDS

1. *Health Care Worker Needlestick Prevention Act* (PL 106-430).

2. *Occupational Exposure to Bloodborne Pathogens: Final Rule.* (OSHA 29 CFR Part 1910.1030).

3. *Occupational Exposure to Bloodborne Pathogens: Needlesticks and Other Sharps Injuries: Final Rule.* (OSHA 29 CFS Part 1910).

4. Updated U.S. Public Health Service. *Guidelines for the Management of Occupational Exposures to HBV, HCV, and HIV and Recommendations for Postexposure Prophylaxis* (Morbidity and Mortality Weekly, June 29, 2001 / 50(RR-11); 1-42.

APPENDIX B-1

Health Care Worker Needlestick Prevention Act (PL 106-430)

To require changes in the bloodborne pathogens standard in effect under the Occupational Safety and Health Act of 1970.

Be it enacted by the Senate and House of Representatives of the United States of America in Congress assembled,

SECTION 1. SHORT TITLE.

This Act may be cited as the "Needlestick Safety and Prevention Act".

SEC. 2. FINDINGS.

The Congress finds the following:

(1) Numerous workers who are occupationally exposed to bloodborne pathogens have contracted fatal and other serious viruses and diseases, including the human immunodeficiency virus (HIV), hepatitis B, and hepatitis C from exposure to blood and other potentially infectious materials in their workplace.

(2) In 1991 the Occupational Safety and Health Administration issued a standard regulating occupational exposure to bloodborne pathogens, including the human immunodeficiency virus, (HIV), the hepatitis B virus (HBV), and the hepatitis C virus (HCV).

(3) Compliance with the bloodborne pathogens standard has significantly reduced the risk that workers will contract a bloodborne disease in the course of their work.

(4) Nevertheless, occupational exposure to bloodborne pathogens from accidental sharps injuries in health care settings continues to be a serious problem. In March 2000, the Centers for Disease Control and Prevention estimated that more than 380,000 percutaneous injuries from contaminated sharps occur annually among health care workers in United States hospital settings. Estimates for all health care settings are that 600,000 to 800,000 needlestick and other percutaneous injuries occur among health care workers annually. Such injuries can involve needles or other sharps contaminated with bloodborne pathogens, such as HIV, HBV, or HCV.

(5) Since publication of the bloodborne pathogens standard in 1991 there has been a substantial increase in the number and assortment of effective engineering controls available to employers. There is now a large body of research and data concerning the effectiveness of newer engineering controls, including safer medical devices.

(6) 396 interested parties responded to a Request for Information (in this section referred to as the "RFI") conducted by the Occupational Safety and Health Administration in 1998 on engineering and work practice controls used to eliminate or minimize the risk of occupational exposure to bloodborne pathogens due to percutaneous injuries from contaminated sharps. Comments were provided by health care facilities, groups representing healthcare workers, researchers, educational institutions, professional and industry associations, and manufacturers of medical devices.

(7) Numerous studies have demonstrated that the use of safer medical devices, such as needleless systems and sharps with engineered sharps injury protections, when they are part of an overall bloodborne pathogens risk-reduction program, can be extremely effective in reducing accidental sharps injuries.

(8) In March 2000, the Centers for Disease Control and Prevention estimated that, depending on the type of device used and the procedure involved, 62 to 88 percent of sharps injuries can potentially be prevented by the use of safer medical devices.

(9) The OSHA 200 Log, as it is currently maintained, does not sufficiently reflect injuries that may involve exposure to bloodborne pathogens in healthcare facilities. More than 98 percent of healthcare facilities responding to the RFI have adopted surveillance systems in addition to the OSHA 200 Log. Information gathered through these surveillance systems is commonly used for hazard identification and evaluation of program and device effectiveness.

(10) Training and education in the use of safer medical devices and safer work practices are significant elements in the prevention of percutaneous exposure incidents. Staff involvement in the device selection and evaluation process is also an important element to achieving a reduction in sharps injuries, particularly as new safer devices are introduced into the work setting.

(11) Modification of the bloodborne pathogens standard is appropriate to set forth in greater detail its requirement that employers identify, evaluate, and make use of effective safer medical devices.

SEC. 3. BLOODBORNE PATHOGENS STANDARD.

The bloodborne pathogens standard published at 29 CFR 1910.1030 shall be revised as follows:

(1) The definition of "Engineering Controls" (at 29 CFR 1910.1030(b)) shall include as additional examples of controls the following: ``safer medical devices, such as sharps with engineered sharps injury protections and needleless systems''.

(2) The term "Sharps with Engineered Sharps Injury Protections" shall be added to the definitions (at 29 CFR 1910.1030(b)) and defined as ``a nonneedle sharp or a needle device used for withdrawing body fluids, accessing a vein or artery, or administering medications or other fluids, with a built-in safety feature or mechanism that effectively reduces the risk of an exposure incident''.

(3) The term "Needleless Systems" shall be added to the definitions (at 29 CFR 1910.1030(b)) and defined as "a device that does not use needles for: (A) the collection of bodily fluids or withdrawal of body fluids after initial venous or arterial access is established; (B) the administration of medication or fluids; or (C) any other procedure involving the potential for occupational exposure to bloodborne pathogens due to percutaneous injuries from contaminated sharps".

(4) In addition to the existing requirements concerning exposure control plans (29 CFR 1910.1030(c)(1)(iv)), the review and update of such plans shall be required to also--

(A) "reflect changes in technology that eliminate or reduce exposure to bloodborne pathogens"; and

(B) "document annually consideration and implementation of appropriate commercially available and effective safer medical devices designed to eliminate or minimize occupational exposure".

(5) The following additional recordkeeping requirement shall be added to the bloodborne pathogens standard at 29 CFR 1910.1030(h): "The employer shall establish and maintain a sharps injury log for the recording of percutaneous injuries from contaminated sharps. The information in the sharps injury log shall be recorded and maintained in such manner as to protect the confidentiality of the injured employee. The sharps injury log shall contain, at a minimum--

(A) the type and brand of device involved in the incident,

(B) the department or work area where the exposure incident occurred, and

(C) an explanation of how the incident occurred".

The requirement for such sharps injury log shall not apply to any employer who is not required to maintain a log of occupational injuries and illnesses under 29 CFR 1904 and the sharps injury log shall be maintained for the period required by 29 CFR 1904.6.

(6) The following new section shall be added to the bloodborne pathogens standard: "An employer, who is required to establish an Exposure Control Plan shall solicit input from non-managerial employees responsible for direct patient care who are potentially exposed to injuries from contaminated sharps in the identification, evaluation, and selection of effective engineering and work practice controls and shall document the solicitation in the Exposure Control Plan".

SEC. 4. EFFECT OF MODIFICATIONS.

The modifications under section 3 shall be in force until superseded in whole or in part by regulations promulgated by the Secretary of Labor under section 6(b) of the Occupational Safety and Health Act of 1970 (29 U.S.C. 655(b)) and shall be enforced in the same manner and to the same extent as any rule or regulation promulgated under section 6(b).

SEC. 5. PROCEDURE AND EFFECTIVE DATE.

(a) Procedure --The modifications of the bloodborne pathogens standard prescribed by section 3 shall take effect without regard to the procedural requirements applicable to regulations promulgated under section 6(b) of the Occupational Safety and Health Act of 1970 (29 U.S.C. 655(b)) or the procedural requirements of chapter 5 of title 5, United States Code.

(b) Effective Date --The modifications to the bloodborne pathogens standard required by section 3 shall--

(1) within 6 months of the date of the enactment of this Act, be made and published in the Federal Register by the Secretary of Labor acting through the Occupational Safety and Health Administration; and

(2) at the end of 90 days after such publication, take effect.

APPENDIX B-2

DEPARTMENT OF LABOR, OCCUPATIONAL SAFETY and HEALTH ADMINISTRATION 29 CFR part 1910.1030, SubPart: Z: Occupational Exposure to Bloodborne Pathogens (Final Rule)

(a) *Scope and Application.* This section applies to all occupational exposure to blood or other potentially infectious materials as defined by paragraph (b) of this section.

(b) *Definitions.* For purposes of this section, the following shall apply:

Assistant Secretary means the Assistant Secretary of Labor for Occupational Safety and Health, or designated representative.

Blood means human blood, human blood components, and products made from human blood.

Bloodborne Pathogens means pathogenic microorganisms that are present in human blood and can cause disease in humans. These pathogens include, but are not limited to, hepatitis B virus (HBV) and human immunodeficiency virus (HIV).

Clinical Laboratory means a workplace where diagnostic or other screening procedures are performed on blood or other potentially infectious materials.

Contaminated means the presence or the reasonably anticipated presence of blood or other potentially infectious materials on an item or surface.

Contaminated Laundry means laundry which has been soiled with blood or other potentially infectious materials or may contain sharps.

Contaminated Sharps means any contaminated object that can penetrate the skin including, but not limited to, needles, scalpels, broken glass, broken capillary tubes, and exposed ends of dental wires.

Decontamination means the use of physical or chemical means to remove, inactivate, or destroy bloodborne pathogens on a surface or item to the point where they are no longer capable of transmitting infectious particles and the surface or item is rendered safe for handling, use, or disposal.

Director means the Director of the National Institute for Occupational Safety and Health, U.S. Department of Health and Human Services, or designated representative.

Engineering Controls means controls (e.g., sharps disposal containers, self-sheathing needles) that isolate or remove the bloodborne pathogens hazard from the workplace.

Exposure Incident means a specific eye, mouth, other mucous membrane, non-intact skin, or parenteral contact with blood or other potentially infectious materials that results from the performance of an employee's duties.

Handwashing Facilities means a facility providing an adequate supply of running potable water, soap and single use towels or hot air drying machines.

Licensed Healthcare Professional is a person whose legally permitted scope of practice allows him or her to independently perform the activities required by paragraph (f) Hepatitis B Vaccination and Post-exposure Evaluation and Follow-up.

HBV means hepatitis B virus.

HIV means human immunodeficiency virus.

Occupational Exposure means reasonably anticipated skin, eye, mucous membrane, or parenteral contact with blood or other potentially infectious materials that may result from the performance of an employee's duties.

Other Potentially Infectious Materials means (1) The following human body fluids: semen, vaginal secretions, cerebrospinal fluid, synovial fluid, pleural fluid, pericardial fluid, peritoneal fluid, amniotic fluid, saliva in dental procedures, any body fluid that is visibly contaminated with blood, and all body fluids in situations where it is difficult or impossible to differentiate between body fluids; (2) Any unfixed tissue or organ (other than intact skin) from a human (living or dead); and (3) HIV-containing cell or tissue cultures, organ cultures, and HIV- or HBV-containing culture medium or other solutions; and blood, organs, or other tissues from experimental animals infected with HIV or HBV.

Parenteral means piercing mucous membranes or the skin barrier through such events as needlesticks, human bites, cuts, and abrasions.

Personal Protective Equipment is specialized clothing or equipment worn by an employee for protection against a hazard. General work clothes (e.g., uniforms, pants, shirts or blouses) not intended to function as protection against a hazard are not considered to be personal protective equipment.

Production Facility means a facility engaged in industrial-scale, large-volume or high concentration production of HIV or HBV.

Regulated Waste means liquid or semi-liquid blood or other potentially infectious materials; contaminated items that would release blood or other potentially infectious materials in a liquid or semi-liquid state if compressed; items that are caked with dried blood or other potentially infectious materials and are capable of releasing these materials during handling; contaminated sharps; and pathological and microbiological wastes containing blood or other potentially infectious materials.

Research Laboratory means a laboratory producing or using research-laboratory-scale amounts of HIV or HBV. Research laboratories may produce high concentrations of HIV or HBV but not in the volume found in production facilities.

Source Individual means any individual, living or dead, whose blood or other potentially infectious materials may be a source of occupational exposure to the employee. Examples include, but are not limited to, hospital and clinic patients; clients in institutions for the developmentally disabled; trauma victims; clients of drug and alcohol treatment facilities; residents of hospices and nursing homes; human remains; and individuals who donate or sell blood or blood components.

Sterilize means the use of a physical or chemical procedure to destroy all microbial life including highly resistant bacterial endospores.

Universal Precautions is an approach to infection control. According to the concept of Universal Precautions, all human blood and certain human body fluids are treated as if known to be infectious for HIV, HBV, and other bloodborne pathogens.

Work Practice Controls means controls that reduce the likelihood of exposure by altering the manner in which a task is performed (e.g., prohibiting recapping of needles by a two-handed technique).

(c) Exposure Control.

(c)(1) Exposure Control Plan.

(c)(1)(i) Each employer having an employee(s) with occupational exposure as defined by paragraph (b) of this section shall establish a written Exposure Control Plan designed to eliminate or minimize employee exposure.

(c)(1)(ii) The Exposure Control Plan shall contain at least the following elements:

(c)(1)(ii)(A) The exposure determination required by paragraph (c)(2),

(c)(1)(ii)(B) The schedule and method of implementation for paragraphs (d) Methods of Compliance, (e) HIV and HBV Research Laboratories and Production Facilities, (f) Hepatitis B Vaccination and Post-Exposure Evaluation and Follow-up, (g) Communication of Hazards to Employees, and (h) Recordkeeping, of this standard, and

(c)(1)(ii)(C) The procedure for the evaluation of circumstances surrounding exposure incidents as required by paragraph (f)(3)(i) of this standard.

(c)(1)(iii) Each employer shall ensure that a copy of the Exposure Control Plan is accessible to employees in accordance with 29 CFR 1910.1020(e).

(c)(1)(iv) The Exposure Control Plan shall be reviewed and updated at least annually and whenever necessary to reflect new or modified tasks and procedures which affect occupational exposure and to reflect new or revised employee positions with occupational exposure.

(c)(1)(v) The Exposure Control Plan shall be made available to the Assistant Secretary and the Director upon request for examination and copying.

(c)(2) Exposure Determination.

(c)(2)(i) Each employer who has an employee(s) with occupational exposure as defined by paragraph (b) of this section shall prepare an exposure determination. This exposure determination shall contain the following:

(c)(2)(i)(A) A list of all job classifications in which all employees in those job classifications have occupational exposure;

 (c)(2)(i)(B) A list of job classifications in which some employees have occupational exposure, and

(c)(2)(i)(C) A list of all tasks and procedures or groups of closely related task and procedures in which occupational exposure occurs and that are performed by employees in job classifications listed in accordance with the provisions of paragraph (c)(2)(i)(B) of this standard.

(c)(2)(ii) This exposure determination shall be made without regard to the use of personal protective equipment.

(d) Methods of Compliance.

(d)(1) General. Universal precautions shall be observed to prevent contact with blood or other potentially infectious materials. Under circumstances in which differentiation between body fluid types is difficult or impossible, all body fluids shall be considered potentially infectious materials.

(d)(2) Engineering and Work Practice Controls.

(d)(2)(i) Engineering and work practice controls shall be used to eliminate or minimize employee exposure. Where occupational exposure remains after institution of these controls, personal protective equipment shall also be used.

(d)(2)(ii) Engineering controls shall be examined and maintained or replaced on a regular schedule to ensure their effectiveness.

(d)(2)(iii) Employers shall provide handwashing facilities which are readily accessible to employees.

(d)(2)(iv) When provision of handwashing facilities is not feasible, the employer shall provide either an appropriate antiseptic hand cleanser in conjunction with clean cloth/paper towels or antiseptic towelettes. When antiseptic hand cleansers or towelettes are used, hands shall be washed with soap and running water as soon as feasible.

(d)(2)(v) Employers shall ensure that employees wash their hands immediately or as soon as feasible after removal of gloves or other personal protective equipment.

(d)(2)(vi) Employers shall ensure that employees wash hands and any other skin with soap and water, or flush mucous membranes with water immediately or as soon as feasible following contact of such body areas with blood or other potentially infectious materials.

(d)(2)(vii) Contaminated needles and other contaminated sharps shall not be bent, recapped, or removed except as noted in paragraphs (d)(2)(vii)(A) and (d)(2)(vii)(B) below. Shearing or breaking of contaminated needles is prohibited.

(d)(2)(vii)(A) Contaminated needles and other contaminated sharps shall not be bent, recapped or removed unless the employer can demonstrate that no alternative is feasible or that such action is required by a specific medical or dental procedure.

(d)(2)(vii)(B) Such bending, recapping or needle removal must be accomplished through the use of a mechanical device or a one-handed technique.

(d)(2)(viii) Immediately or as soon as possible after use, contaminated reusable sharps shall be placed in appropriate containers until properly reprocessed. These containers shall be:

(d)(2)(viii)(A) puncture resistant;

(d)(2)(viii)(B) labeled or color-coded in accordance with this standard;

(d)(2)(viii)(C) leakproof on the sides and bottom; and

(d)(2)(viii)(D) in accordance with the requirements set forth in paragraph(d)(4)(ii)(E) for reusable sharps.

(d)(2)(ix) Eating, drinking, smoking, applying cosmetics or lip balm, and handling contact lenses are prohibited in work areas where there is a reasonable likelihood of occupational exposure.

(d)(2)(x) Food and drink shall not be kept in refrigerators, freezers, shelves, cabinets or on countertops or benchtops where blood or other potentially infectious materials are present.

(d)(2)(xi) All procedures involving blood or other potentially infectious materials shall be performed in such a manner as to minimize splashing, spraying, spattering, and generation of droplets of these substances.

(d)(2)(xii) Mouth pipetting/suctioning of blood or other potentially infectious materials is prohibited.

(d)(2)(xiii) Specimens of blood or other potentially infectious materials shall be placed in a container which prevents leakage during collection, handling, processing, storage, transport, or shipping.

(d)(2)(xiii)(A) The container for storage, transport, or shipping shall be labeled or color-coded according to paragraph (g)(1)(i) and closed prior to being stored, transported, or shipped. When a facility utilizes Universal Precautions in the handling of all specimens, the labeling/color-coding of specimens is not necessary provided containers are recognizable as containing specimens. This exemption only applies while such specimens/containers remain within the facility. Labeling or color-coding in accordance with paragraph (g)(1)(i) is required when such specimens/containers leave the facility.

(d)(2)(xiii)(B) If outside contamination of the primary container occurs, the primary container shall be placed within a second container which prevents leakage during handling, processing, storage, transport, or shipping and is labeled or color-coded according to the requirements of this standard.

(d)(2)(xiii)(C) If the specimen could puncture the primary container, the primary container shall be placed within a secondary container which is puncture-resistant in addition to the above characteristics.

(d)(2)(xiv) Equipment which may become contaminated with blood or other potentially infectious materials shall be examined prior to servicing or shipping and shall be decontaminated as necessary, unless the employer can demonstrate that decontamination of such equipment or portions of such equipment is not feasible.

(d)(2)(xiv)(A) A readily observable label in accordance with paragraph (g)(1)(i)(H) shall be attached to the equipment stating which portions remain contaminated.

(d)(2)(xiv)(B) The employer shall ensure that this information is conveyed to all affected employees, the servicing representative, and/or the manufacturer, as appropriate, prior to handling, servicing, or shipping so that appropriate precautions will be taken.

(d)(3) Personal Protective Equipment.

(d)(3)(i) Provision. When there is occupational exposure, the employer shall provide, at no cost to the employee, appropriate personal protective equipment such as, but not limited to, gloves, gowns, laboratory coats, face shields or masks and eye protection, and mouthpieces, resuscitation bags, pocket masks, or other ventilation devices. Personal protective equipment will be considered "appropriate" only if it does not permit blood or other potentially infectious materials to pass through to or reach the employee's work clothes, street clothes, undergarments, skin, eyes, mouth, or other mucous membranes under normal conditions of use and for the duration of time which the protective equipment will be used.

(d)(3)(ii) Use. The employer shall ensure that the employee uses appropriate personal protective equipment unless the employer shows that the employee temporarily and briefly declined to use personal protective equipment when, under rare and extraordinary circumstances, it was the employee's professional judgment that in the specific instance its use would have prevented the delivery of health care or public safety services or would have posed an increased hazard to the safety of the worker or co-worker. When the employee makes this judgement, the circumstances shall be investigated and documented in order to determine whether changes can be instituted to prevent such occurrences in the future.

(d)(3)(iii) Accessibility. The employer shall ensure that appropriate personal protective equipment in the appropriate sizes is readily accessible at the worksite or is issued to employees. Hypoallergenic gloves, glove liners, powderless gloves, or other similar alternatives shall be readily accessible to those employees who are allergic to the gloves normally provided.

(d)(3)(iv) Cleaning, Laundering, and Disposal. The employer shall clean, launder, and dispose of personal protective equipment required by paragraphs (d) and (e) of this standard, at no cost to the employee.

(d)(3)(v) Repair and Replacement. The employer shall repair or replace personal protective equipment as needed to maintain its effectiveness, at no cost to the employee.

(d)(3)(vi) If a garment(s) is penetrated by blood or other potentially infectious materials, the garment(s) shall be removed immediately or as soon as feasible.

(d)(3)(vii) All personal protective equipment shall be removed prior to leaving the work area.

(d)(3)(viii) When personal protective equipment is removed it shall be placed in an appropriately designated area or container for storage, washing, decontamination or disposal.

(d)(3)(ix) Gloves. Gloves shall be worn when it can be reasonably anticipated that the employee may have hand contact with blood, other potentially infectious materials, mucous membranes, and non-intact skin; when performing vascular access procedures except as specified in paragraph (d)(3)(ix)(D); and when handling or touching contaminated items or surfaces.

(d)(3)(ix)(A) Disposable (single use) gloves such as surgical or examination gloves, shall be replaced as soon as practical when contaminated or as soon as feasible if they are torn, punctured, or when their ability to function as a barrier is compromised.

(d)(3)(ix)(B) Disposable (single use) gloves shall not be washed or decontaminated for re-use.

(d)(3)(ix)(C) Utility gloves may be decontaminated for re-use if the integrity of the glove is not compromised. However, they must be discarded if they are cracked, peeling, torn, punctured, or exhibit other signs of deterioration or when their ability to function as a barrier is compromised.

(d)(3)(ix)(D) If an employer in a volunteer blood donation center judges that routine gloving for all phlebotomies is not necessary then the employer shall:

(d)(3)(ix)(D)(1) Periodically reevaluate this policy;

(d)(3)(ix)(D)(2) Make gloves available to all employees who wish to use them for phlebotomy;

(d)(3)(ix)(D)(3) Not discourage the use of gloves for phlebotomy; and

(d)(3)(ix)(D)(4) Require that gloves be used for phlebotomy in the following circumstances:

[i] When the employee has cuts, scratches, or other breaks in his or her skin;

[ii] When the employee judges that hand contamination with blood may occur, for example, when performing phlebotomy on an uncooperative source individual; and

[iii] When the employee is receiving training in phlebotomy.

(d)(3)(x) Masks, Eye Protection, and Face Shields. Masks in combination with eye protection devices, such as goggles or glasses with solid side shields, or chin-length face shields, shall be worn whenever splashes, spray, spatter, or droplets of blood or other potentially infectious materials may be generated and eye, nose, or mouth contamination can be reasonably anticipated.

(d)(3)(xi) Gowns, Aprons, and Other Protective Body Clothing. Appropriate protective clothing such as, but not limited to, gowns, aprons, lab coats, clinic jackets, or similar outer garments shall be worn in occupational exposure situations. The type and characteristics will depend upon the task and degree of exposure anticipated.

(d)(3)(xii) Surgical caps or hoods and/or shoe covers or boots shall be worn in instances when gross contamination can reasonably be anticipated (e.g., autopsies, orthopaedic surgery).

(d)(4) Housekeeping.

(d)(4)(i) General. Employers shall ensure that the worksite is maintained in a clean and sanitary condition. The employer shall determine and implement an appropriate written schedule for cleaning and method of decontamination based upon the location within the facility, type of surface to be cleaned, type of soil present, and tasks or procedures being performed in the area.

(d)(4)(ii) All equipment and environmental and working surfaces shall be cleaned and decontaminated after contact with blood or other potentially infectious materials.

(d)(4)(ii)(A) Contaminated work surfaces shall be decontaminated with an appropriate disinfectant after completion of procedures; immediately or as soon as feasible when surfaces are overtly contaminated or after any spill of blood or other potentially infectious materials; and at the end of the work shift if the surface may have become contaminated since the last cleaning.

(d)(4)(ii)(B) Protective coverings, such as plastic wrap, aluminum foil, or imperviously-backed absorbent paper used to cover equipment and environmental surfaces, shall be removed and replaced as soon as feasible when they become overtly contaminated or at the end of the workshift if they may have become contaminated during the shift.

(d)(4)(ii)(C) All bins, pails, cans, and similar receptacles intended for reuse which have a reasonable likelihood for becoming contaminated with blood or other potentially infectious materials shall be inspected and decontaminated on a regularly scheduled basis and cleaned and decontaminated immediately or as soon as feasible upon visible contamination.

(d)(4)(ii)(D) Broken glassware which may be contaminated shall not be picked up directly with the hands. It shall be cleaned up using mechanical means, such as a brush and dust pan, tongs, or forceps.

(d)(4)(ii)(E) Reusable sharps that are contaminated with blood or other potentially infectious materials shall not be stored or processed in a manner that requires employees to reach by hand into the containers where these sharps have been placed.

(d)(4)(iii) Regulated Waste.

(d)(4)(iii)(A) Contaminated Sharps Discarding and Containment.

(d)(4)(iii)(A)(1) Contaminated sharps shall be discarded immediately or as soon as feasible in containers that are:

[a] Closable;

[b] Puncture resistant;

[c] Leakproof on sides and bottom; and

[d] Labeled or color-coded in accordance with paragraph (g)(1)(i) of this standard.

(d)(4)(iii)(A)(2) During use, containers for contaminated sharps shall be:

[a] Easily accessible to personnel and located as close as is feasible to the immediate area where sharps are used or can be reasonably anticipated to be found (e.g., laundries);

[b] Maintained upright throughout use; and

[c] Replaced routinely and not be allowed to overfill.

(d)(4)(iii)(A)(3) When moving containers of contaminated sharps from the area of use, the containers shall be:

[a] Closed immediately prior to removal or replacement to prevent spillage or protrusion of contents during handling, storage, transport, or shipping;

[b] Placed in a secondary container if leakage is possible. The second container shall be:

[i] Closable;

[ii] Constructed to contain all contents and prevent leakage during handling, storage, transport, or shipping; and

[iii] Labeled or color-coded according to paragraph (g)(1)(i) of this standard.

(d)(4)(iii)(A)(4) Reusable containers shall not be opened, emptied, or cleaned manually or in any other manner which would expose employees to the risk of percutaneous injury.

(d)(4)(iii)(B) Other Regulated Waste Containment.

(d)(4)(iii)(B)(1) Regulated waste shall be placed in containers which are:

[a] Closable;

[b] Constructed to contain all contents and prevent leakage of fluids during handling, storage, transport or shipping;

[c] Labeled or color-coded in accordance with paragraph (g)(1)(i) this standard; and

[d] Closed prior to removal to prevent spillage or protrusion of contents during handling, storage, transport, or shipping.

(d)(4)(iii)(B)(2) If outside contamination of the regulated waste container occurs, it shall be placed in a second container. The second container shall be:

[a] Closable;

[b] Constructed to contain all contents and prevent leakage of fluids during handling, storage, transport or shipping;

[c] Labeled or color-coded in accordance with paragraph (g)(1)(i) of this standard; and

[d] Closed prior to removal to prevent spillage or protrusion of contents during handling, storage, transport, or shipping.

(d)(4)(iii)(C) Disposal of all regulated waste shall be in accordance with applicable regulations of the United States, States and Territories, and political subdivisions of States and Territories.

(d)(4)(iv) Laundry.

(d)(4)(iv)(A) Contaminated laundry shall be handled as little as possible with a minimum of agitation.

(d)(4)(iv)(A)(1) Contaminated laundry shall be bagged or containerized at the location where it was used and shall not be sorted or rinsed in the location of use.

(d)(4)(iv)(A)(2) Contaminated laundry shall be placed and transported in bags or containers labeled or color-coded in accordance with paragraph (g)(1)(i) of this standard. When a facility utilizes Universal Precautions in the handling of all soiled laundry, alternative labeling or color-coding is sufficient if it permits all employees to recognize the containers as requiring compliance with Universal Precautions.

(d)(4)(iv)(A)(3) Whenever contaminated laundry is wet and presents a reasonable likelihood of soak-through of or leakage from the bag or container, the laundry shall be placed and transported in bags or containers which prevent soak-through and/or leakage of fluids to the exterior.

(d)(4)(iv)(B) The employer shall ensure that employees who have contact with contaminated laundry wear protective gloves and other appropriate personal protective equipment.

(d)(4)(iv)(C) When a facility ships contaminated laundry off-site to a second facility which does not utilize Universal Precautions in the handling of all laundry, the facility generating the contaminated laundry must place such laundry in bags or containers which are labeled or color-coded in accordance with paragraph (g)(1)(i).

(e) HIV and HBV Research Laboratories and Production Facilities.

(e)(1) This paragraph applies to research laboratories and production facilities engaged in the culture, production, concentration, experimentation, and manipulation of HIV and HBV. It does not apply to clinical or diagnostic laboratories engaged solely in the analysis of blood, tissues, or organs. These requirements apply in addition to the other requirements of the standard.

(e)(2) Research laboratories and production facilities shall meet the following criteria:

(e)(2)(i) Standard Microbiological Practices. All regulated waste shall either be incinerated or decontaminated by a method such as autoclaving known to effectively destroy bloodborne pathogens.

(e)(2)(ii) Special Practices

(e)(2)(ii)(A) Laboratory doors shall be kept closed when work involving HIV or HBV is in progress.

(e)(2)(ii)(B) Contaminated materials that are to be decontaminated at a site away from the work area shall be placed in a durable, leakproof, labeled or color-coded container that is closed before being removed from the work area.

(e)(2)(ii)(C) Access to the work area shall be limited to authorized persons. Written policies and procedures shall be established whereby only persons who have been advised of the potential biohazard, who meet any specific entry requirements, and who comply with all entry and exit procedures shall be allowed to enter the work areas and animal rooms.

(e)(2)(ii)(D) When other potentially infectious materials or infected animals are present in the work area or containment module, a hazard warning sign incorporating the universal biohazard symbol shall be posted on all access doors. The hazard warning sign shall comply with paragraph (g)(1)(ii) of this standard.

(e)(2)(ii)(E) All activities involving other potentially infectious materials shall be conducted in biological safety cabinets or other physical-containment devices within the containment module. No work with these other potentially infectious materials shall be conducted on the open bench.

(e)(2)(ii)(F) Laboratory coats, gowns, smocks, uniforms, or other appropriate protective clothing shall be used in the work area and animal rooms. Protective clothing shall not be worn outside of the work area and shall be decontaminated before being laundered.

(e)(2)(ii)(G) Special care shall be taken to avoid skin contact with other potentially infectious materials. Gloves shall be worn when handling infected animals and when making hand contact with other potentially infectious materials is unavoidable.

(e)(2)(ii)(H) Before disposal all waste from work areas and from animal rooms shall either be incinerated or decontaminated by a method such as autoclaving known to effectively destroy bloodborne pathogens.

(e)(2)(ii)(I) Vacuum lines shall be protected with liquid disinfectant traps and high-efficiency particulate air (HEPA) filters or filters of equivalent or superior efficiency and which are checked routinely and maintained or replaced as necessary.

(e)(2)(ii)(J) Hypodermic needles and syringes shall be used only for parenteral injection and aspiration of fluids from laboratory animals and diaphragm bottles. Only needle-locking syringes or disposable syringe-needle units (i.e., the needle is integral to the syringe) shall be used for the injection or aspiration of other potentially infectious materials. Extreme caution shall be used when handling needles and syringes. A needle shall not be bent, sheared, replaced in the sheath or guard, or removed from the syringe following use. The needle and syringe shall be promptly placed in a puncture-resistant container and autoclaved or decontaminated before reuse or disposal.

(e)(2)(ii)(K) All spills shall be immediately contained and cleaned up by appropriate professional staff or others properly trained and equipped to work with potentially concentrated infectious materials.

(e)(2)(ii)(L) A spill or accident that results in an exposure incident shall be immediately reported to the laboratory director or other responsible person.

(e)(2)(ii)(M) A biosafety manual shall be prepared or adopted and periodically reviewed and updated at least annually or more often if necessary. Personnel shall be advised of potential hazards, shall be required to read instructions on practices and procedures, and shall be required to follow them.

(e)(2)(iii) Containment Equipment.

(e)(2)(iii)(A) Certified biological safety cabinets (Class I, II, or III) or other appropriate combinations of personal protection or physical containment devices, such as special protective clothing, respirators, centrifuge safety cups, sealed centrifuge rotors, and containment caging for animals, shall be used for all activities with other potentially infectious materials that pose a threat of exposure to droplets, splashes, spills, or aerosols.

(e)(2)(iii)(B) Biological safety cabinets shall be certified when installed, whenever they are moved and at least annually.

(e)(3) HIV and HBV research laboratories shall meet the following criteria:

(e)(3)(i) Each laboratory shall contain a facility for hand washing and an eye wash facility which is readily available within the work area.

(e)(3)(ii) An autoclave for decontamination of regulated waste shall be available.

(e)(4) HIV and HBV production facilities shall meet the following criteria:

(e)(4)(i) The work areas shall be separated from areas that are open to unrestricted traffic flow within the building. Passage through two sets of doors shall be the basic requirement for entry into the work area from access corridors or other contiguous areas. Physical separation of the high-containment work area from access corridors or other areas or activities may also be provided by a double-doored clothes-change room (showers may be included), airlock, or other access facility that requires passing through two sets of doors before entering the work area.

(e)(4)(ii) The surfaces of doors, walls, floors and ceilings in the work area shall be water resistant so that they can be easily cleaned. Penetrations in these surfaces shall be sealed or capable of being sealed to facilitate decontamination.

(e)(4)(iii) Each work area shall contain a sink for washing hands and a readily available eye wash facility. The sink shall be foot, elbow, or automatically operated and shall be located near the exit door of the work area.

(e)(4)(iv) Access doors to the work area or containment module shall be self-closing.

(e)(4)(v) An autoclave for decontamination of regulated waste shall be available within or as near as possible to the work area.

(e)(4)(vi) A ducted exhaust-air ventilation system shall be provided. This system shall create directional airflow that draws air into the work area through the entry area. The exhaust air shall not be recirculated to any other area of the building, shall be discharged to the outside, and shall be dispersed away from occupied areas and air intakes. The proper direction of the airflow shall be verified (i.e., into the work area).

(e)(5) Training Requirements. Additional training requirements for employees in HIV and HBV research laboratories and HIV and HBV production facilities are specified in paragraph (g)(2)(ix).

(f) Hepatitis B Vaccination and Post-exposure Evaluation and Follow-up.

(f)(1) General.

(f)(1)(i) The employer shall make available the hepatitis B vaccine and vaccination series to all employees who have occupational exposure, and post-exposure evaluation and follow-up to all employees who have had an exposure incident.

(f)(1)(ii) The employer shall ensure that all medical evaluations and procedures including the hepatitis B vaccine and vaccination series and post-exposure evaluation and follow-up, including prophylaxis, are:

(f)(1)(ii)(A) Made available at no cost to the employee;

(f)(1)(ii)(B) Made available to the employee at a reasonable time and place;

(f)(1)(ii)(C) Performed by or under the supervision of a licensed physician or by or under the supervision of another licensed healthcare professional; and

(f)(1)(ii)(D) Provided according to recommendations of the U.S. Public Health Service current at the time these evaluations and procedures take place, except as specified by this paragraph (f).

(f)(1)(iii) The employer shall ensure that all laboratory tests are conducted by an accredited laboratory at no cost to the employee.

(f)(2) Hepatitis B Vaccination.

(f)(2)(i) Hepatitis B vaccination shall be made available after the employee has received the training required in paragraph (g)(2)(vii)(I) and within 10 working days of initial assignment to all employees who have occupational exposure unless the employee has previously received the complete hepatitis B vaccination series, antibody testing has revealed that the employee is immune, or the vaccine is contraindicated for medical reasons.

(f)(2)(ii) The employer shall not make participation in a prescreening program a prerequisite for receiving hepatitis B vaccination.

(f)(2)(iii) If the employee initially declines hepatitis B vaccination but at a later date while still covered under the standard decides to accept the vaccination, the employer shall make available hepatitis B vaccination at that time.

(f)(2)(iv) The employer shall assure that employees who decline to accept hepatitis B vaccination offered by the employer sign the statement in Appendix A.

(f)(2)(v) If a routine booster dose(s) of hepatitis B vaccine is recommended by the U.S. Public Health Service at a future date, such booster dose(s) shall be made available in accordance with section (f)(1)(ii).

(f)(3) Post-exposure Evaluation and Follow-up. Following a report of an exposure incident, the employer shall make immediately available to the exposed employee a confidential medical evaluation and follow-up, including at least the following elements:

(f)(3)(i) Documentation of the route(s) of exposure, and the circumstances under which the exposure incident occurred;

(f)(3)(ii) Identification and documentation of the source individual, unless the employer can establish that identification is infeasible or prohibited by state or local law;

(f)(3)(ii)(A) The source individual's blood shall be tested as soon as feasible and after consent is obtained in order to determine HBV and HIV infectivity. If consent is not obtained, the employer shall establish that legally required consent cannot be obtained. When the source individual's consent is not required by law, the source individual's blood, if available, shall be tested and the results documented.

(f)(3)(ii)(B) When the source individual is already known to be infected with HBV or HIV, testing for the source individual's known HBV or HIV status need not be repeated.

(f)(3)(ii)(C) Results of the source individual's testing shall be made available to the exposed employee, and the employee shall be informed of applicable laws and regulations concerning disclosure of the identity and infectious status of the source individual.

(f)(3)(iii) Collection and testing of blood for HBV and HIV serological status;

(f)(3)(iii)(A) The exposed employee's blood shall be collected as soon as feasible and tested after consent is obtained.

(f)(3)(iii)(B) If the employee consents to baseline blood collection, but does not give consent at that time for HIV serologic testing, the sample shall be preserved for at least 90 days. If, within 90 days of the exposure incident, the employee elects to have the baseline sample tested, such testing shall be done as soon as feasible.

(f)(3)(iv) Post-exposure prophylaxis, when medically indicated, as recommended by the U.S. Public Health Service;

(f)(3)(v) Counseling; and

(f)(3)(vi) Evaluation of reported illnesses.

(f)(4) Information Provided to the Healthcare Professional.

(f)(4)(i) The employer shall ensure that the healthcare professional responsible for the employee's Hepatitis B vaccination is provided a copy of this regulation.

(f)(4)(ii) The employer shall ensure that the healthcare professional evaluating an employee after an exposure incident is provided the following information:

(f)(4)(ii)(A) A copy of this regulation;

(f)(4)(ii)(B) A description of the exposed employee's duties as they relate to the exposure incident;

(f)(4)(ii)(C) Documentation of the route(s) of exposure and circumstances under which exposure occurred;

(f)(4)(ii)(D) Results of the source individual's blood testing, if available; and

(f)(4)(ii)(E) All medical records relevant to the appropriate treatment of the employee including vaccination status which are the employer's responsibility to maintain.

(f)(5) Healthcare Professional's Written Opinion. The employer shall obtain and provide the employee with a copy of the evaluating healthcare professional's written opinion within 15 days of the completion of the evaluation.

(f)(5)(i) The healthcare professional's written opinion for Hepatitis B vaccination shall be limited to whether Hepatitis B vaccination is indicated for an employee, and if the employee has received such vaccination.

(f)(5)(ii) The healthcare professional's written opinion for post-exposure evaluation and follow-up shall be limited to the following information:

(f)(5)(ii)(A) That the employee has been informed of the results of the evaluation; and

(f)(5)(ii)(B) That the employee has been told about any medical conditions resulting from exposure to blood or other potentially infectious materials which require further evaluation or treatment.

(f)(5)(iii) All other findings or diagnoses shall remain confidential and shall not be included in the written report.

(f)(6) Medical Recordkeeping. Medical records required by this standard shall be maintained in accordance with paragraph (h)(1) of this section.

(g) Communication of Hazards to Employees.

(g)(1) Labels and Signs.

(g)(1)(i) Labels.

(g)(1)(i)(A) Warning labels shall be affixed to containers of regulated waste, refrigerators and freezers containing blood or other potentially infectious material; and other containers used to store, transport or ship blood or other potentially infectious materials, except as provided in paragraph (g)(1)(i)(E), (F) and (G).

(g)(1)(i)(B) Labels required by this section shall include the following legend:

BIOHAZARD

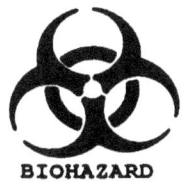

(g)(1)(i)(C) These labels shall be fluorescent orange or orange-red or predominantly so, with lettering and symbols in a contrasting color.

(g)(1)(i)(D) Labels shall be affixed as close as feasible to the container by string, wire, adhesive, or other method that prevents their loss or unintentional removal.

(g)(1)(i)(E) Red bags or red containers may be substituted for labels.

(g)(1)(i)(F) Containers of blood, blood components, or blood products that are labeled as to their contents and have been released for transfusion or other clinical use are exempted from the labeling requirements of paragraph (g).

(g)(1)(i)(G) Individual containers of blood or other potentially infectious materials that are placed in a labeled container during storage, transport, shipment or disposal are exempted from the labeling requirement.

(g)(1)(i)(H) Labels required for contaminated equipment shall be in accordance with this paragraph and shall also state which portions of the equipment remain contaminated.

(g)(1)(i)(I) Regulated waste that has been decontaminated need not be labeled or color-coded.

(g)(1)(ii) Signs.

(g)(1)(ii)(A) The employer shall post signs at the entrance to work areas specified in paragraph (e), HIV and HBV Research Laboratory and Production Facilities, which shall bear the following legend:

BIOHAZARD

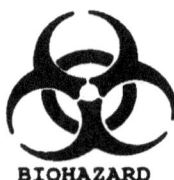

BIOHAZARD

(Name of the Infectious Agent)
(Special requirements for entering the area)
(Name, telephone number of the laboratory director or other
 responsible person.)

(g)(1)(ii)(B) These signs shall be fluorescent orange-red or predominantly so, with lettering and symbols in a contrasting color.

(g)(2) Information and Training.

166

(g)(2)(i) Employers shall ensure that all employees with occupational exposure participate in a training program which must be provided at no cost to the employee and during working hours.

(g)(2)(ii) Training shall be provided as follows:

(g)(2)(ii)(A) At the time of initial assignment to tasks where occupational exposure may take place;

(g)(2)(ii)(B) Within 90 days after the effective date of the standard; and

(g)(2)(ii)(C) At least annually thereafter.

(g)(2)(iii) For employees who have received training on bloodborne pathogens in the year preceding the effective date of the standard, only training with respect to the provisions of the standard which were not included need be provided.

(g)(2)(iv) Annual training for all employees shall be provided within one year of their previous training.

(g)(2)(v) Employers shall provide additional training when changes such as modification of tasks or procedures or institution of new tasks or procedures affect the employee's occupational exposure. The additional training may be limited to addressing the new exposures created.

(g)(2)(vi) Material appropriate in content and vocabulary to educational level, literacy, and language of employees shall be used.

(g)(2)(vii) The training program shall contain at a minimum the following elements:

(g)(2)(vii)(A) An accessible copy of the regulatory text of this standard and an explanation of its contents;

(g)(2)(vii)(B) A general explanation of the epidemiology and symptoms of bloodborne diseases;

(g)(2)(vii)(C) An explanation of the modes of transmission of bloodborne pathogens;

(g)(2)(vii)(D) An explanation of the employer's exposure control plan and the means by which the employee can obtain a copy of the written plan;

(g)(2)(vii)(E) An explanation of the appropriate methods for recognizing tasks and other activities that may involve exposure to blood and other potentially infectious materials;

(g)(2)(vii)(F) An explanation of the use and limitations of methods that will prevent or reduce exposure including appropriate engineering controls, work practices, and personal protective equipment;

(g)(2)(vii)(G) Information on the types, proper use, location, removal, handling, decontamination and disposal of personal protective equipment;

(g)(2)(vii)(H) An explanation of the basis for selection of personal protective equipment;

(g)(2)(vii)(I) Information on the hepatitis B vaccine, including information on its efficacy, safety, method of administration, the benefits of being vaccinated, and that the vaccine and vaccination will be offered free of charge;

(g)(2)(vii)(J) Information on the appropriate actions to take and persons to contact in an emergency involving blood or other potentially infectious materials;

(g)(2)(vii)(K) An explanation of the procedure to follow if an exposure incident occurs, including the method of reporting the incident and the medical follow-up that will be made available;

(g)(2)(vii)(L) Information on the post-exposure evaluation and follow-up that the employer is required to provide for the employee following an exposure incident;

(g)(2)(vii)(M) An explanation of the signs and labels and/or color coding required by paragraph (g)(1); and

(g)(2)(vii)(N) An opportunity for interactive questions and answers with the person conducting the training session.

(g)(2)(viii) The person conducting the training shall be knowledgeable in the subject matter covered by the elements contained in the training program as it relates to the workplace that the training will address.

(g)(2)(ix) Additional Initial Training for Employees in HIV and HBV Laboratories and Production Facilities. Employees in HIV or HBV research laboratories and HIV or HBV production facilities shall receive the following initial training in addition to the above training requirements.

(g)(2)(ix)(A) The employer shall assure that employees demonstrate proficiency in standard microbiological practices and techniques and in the practices and operations specific to the facility before being allowed to work with HIV or HBV.

(g)(2)(ix)(B) The employer shall assure that employees have prior experience in the handling of human pathogens or tissue cultures before working with HIV or HBV.

(g)(2)(ix)(C) The employer shall provide a training program to employees who have no prior experience in handling human pathogens. Initial work activities shall not include the handling of infectious agents. A progression of work activities shall be assigned as techniques are learned and proficiency is developed. The employer shall assure that employees participate in work activities involving infectious agents only after proficiency has been demonstrated.

(h) Recordkeeping.

(h)(1) Medical Records.

(h)(1)(i) The employer shall establish and maintain an accurate record for each employee with occupational exposure, in accordance with 29 CFR 1910.1020.

(h)(1)(ii) This record shall include:

(h)(1)(ii)(A) The name and social security number of the employee;

(h)(1)(ii)(B) A copy of the employee's hepatitis B vaccination status including the dates of all the hepatitis B vaccinations and any medical records relative to the employee's ability to receive vaccination as required by paragraph (f)(2);

(h)(1)(ii)(C) A copy of all results of examinations, medical testing, and follow-up procedures as required by paragraph (f)(3);

(h)(1)(ii)(D) The employer's copy of the healthcare professional's written opinion as required by paragraph (f)(5); and

(h)(1)(ii)(E) A copy of the information provided to the healthcare professional as required by paragraphs (f)(4)(ii)(B)(C) and (D).

(h)(1)(iii) Confidentiality. The employer shall ensure that employee medical records required by paragraph (h)(1) are:

(h)(1)(iii)(A) Kept confidential; and

(h)(1)(iii)(B) Not disclosed or reported without the employee's express written consent to any person within or outside the workplace except as required by this section or as may be required by law.

(h)(1)(iv) The employer shall maintain the records required by paragraph (h) for at least the duration of employment plus 30 years in accordance with 29 CFR 1910.1020.

(h)(2) Training Records.

(h)(2)(i) Training records shall include the following information:

(h)(2)(i)(A) The dates of the training sessions;

(h)(2)(i)(B) The contents or a summary of the training sessions;

(h)(2)(i)(C) The names and qualifications of persons conducting the training; and

(h)(2)(i)(D) The names and job titles of all persons attending the training sessions.

(h)(2)(ii) Training records shall be maintained for 3 years from the date on which the training occurred.

(h)(3) Availability.

(h)(3)(i) The employer shall ensure that all records required to be maintained by this section shall be made available upon request to the Assistant Secretary and the Director for examination and copying.

(h)(3)(ii) Employee training records required by this paragraph shall be provided upon request for examination and copying to employees, to employee representatives, to the Director, and to the Assistant Secretary.

(h)(3)(iii) Employee medical records required by this paragraph shall be provided upon request for examination and copying to the subject employee, to anyone having written consent of the subject employee, to the Director, and to the Assistant Secretary in accordance with 29 CFR 1910.1020.

(h)(4) Transfer of Records.

(h)(4)(i) The employer shall comply with the requirements involving transfer of records set forth in 29 CFR 1910.1020(h).

(h)(4)(ii) If the employer ceases to do business and there is no successor employer to receive and retain the records for the prescribed period, the employer shall notify the Director, at least three months prior to their disposal and transmit them to the Director, if required by the Director to do so, within that three month period.

(i) Dates.

(i)(1) Effective Date. The standard shall become effective on March 6, 1992.

(i)(2) The Exposure Control Plan required by paragraph (c) of this section shall be completed on or before May 5, 1992.

(i)(3) Paragraph (g)(2) Information and Training and (h) Recordkeeping shall take effect on or before June 4, 1992.

(i)(4) Paragraphs (d)(2) Engineering and Work Practice Controls, (d)(3) Personal Protective Equipment, (d)(4) Housekeeping, (e) HIV and HBV Research Laboratories and Production Facilities, (f) Hepatitis B Vaccination and Post-Exposure Evaluation and Follow-up, and (g)(1) Labels and Signs, shall take effect July 6, 1992.

[56 FR 64004, Dec. 06, 1991, as amended at 57 FR 12717, April 13, 1992; 57 FR 29206, July 1, 1992; 61 FR 5507, Feb. 13, 1996]

(NOTE)

Hazardous Waste Operations and Emergency Response Standard

The Hazardous Waste Operations and Emergency Response (HAZWOPER) Standard (29 CFR 1910.120) covers three groups of employees: workers at uncontrolled hazardous waste remediation sites; workers at Resource Conservation Recovery Act (RCRA) permitted hazardous waste treatment, storage, and disposal facilities; and those workers expected to respond to emergencies caused by the uncontrolled release of hazardous substances.

The definition of hazardous substance includes any biological agent or infectious material which may cause disease or death. There are three potential scenarios where the bloodborne and hazardous waste operations and emergency response standard may interface. These scenarios include: workers involved in cleanup operations at hazardous waste sites involving regulated waste; workers at RCRA permitted incinerators that burn infectious waste; and workers responding to an emergency caused by the uncontrolled release of regulated waste (e.g., a transportation accident).

Employers of employees engaged in these three activities must comply with the requirements in 29 CFR 1910.120 as well as the Bloodborne Pathogens Standard. If there is a conflict or overlap, the provision that is more protective of employee health and safety applies.

APPENDIX B-3

DEPARTMENT OF LABOR, OCCUPATIONAL SAFETY and HEALTH ADMINISTRATION 29 CFR part 1910.1030, Occupational Exposure to Bloodborne Pathogens; Needlesticks and Other Sharps Injuries; Final Rule

§ 1910.1030 Bloodborne Pathogens

(a) **Scope and Application**. This section applies to all occupational exposure to blood or other potentially infectious materials as defined by paragraph (b) of this section.

(b) **Definitions**. For purposes of this section, the following shall apply:

Assistant Secretary means the Assistant Secretary of Labor for Occupational Safety and Health, or designated representative.

Blood means human blood, human blood components, and products made from human blood.

Bloodborne Pathogens means pathogenic microorganisms that are present in human blood and can cause disease in humans. These pathogens include, but are not limited to, hepatitis B virus (HBV) and human immunodeficiency virus (HIV).

Clinical Laboratory means a workplace where diagnostic or other screening procedures are performed on blood or other potentially infectious materials.

Contaminated means the presence or the reasonably anticipated presence of blood or other potentially infectious materials on an item or surface.

Contaminated Laundry means laundry which has been soiled with blood or other potentially infectious materials or may contain sharps.

Contaminated Sharps means any contaminated object that can penetrate the skin including, but not limited to, needles, scalpels, broken glass, broken capillary tubes, and exposed ends of dental wires.

Decontamination means the use of physical or chemical means to remove, inactivate, or destroy bloodborne pathogens on a surface or item to the point where they are no longer capable of transmitting infectious particles and the surface or item is rendered safe for handling, use, or disposal.

Director means the Director of the National Institute for Occupational Safety and Health, U.S. Department of Health and Human Services, or designated representative.

Engineering Controls means controls (e.g., sharps disposal containers, self-sheathing needles, safer medical devices, such as sharps with engineered sharps injury protections and needleless systems) that isolate or remove the bloodborne pathogens hazard from the workplace.

Exposure Incident means a specific eye, mouth, other mucous membrane, non-intact skin, or parenteral contact with blood or other potentially infectious materials that results from the performance of an employee's duties.

Handwashing Facilities means a facility providing an adequate supply of running potable water, soap and single use towels or hot air drying machines.

Licensed Healthcare Professional is a person whose legally permitted scope of practice allows him or her to independently perform the activities required by paragraph (f) Hepatitis B Vaccination and Post-exposure Evaluation and Follow-up.

HBV means hepatitis B virus.

HIV means human immunodeficiency virus.

Needleless Systems means a device that does not use needles for (1) the collection of bodily fluids or withdrawal of body fluids after initial venous or arterial access is established; (2) the administration of medication or fluids; or (3) any other procedure involving the potential for occupational exposure to bloodborne pathogens due to percutaneous injuries from contaminated sharps.

Occupational Exposure means reasonably anticipated skin, eye, mucous membrane, or parenteral contact with blood or other potentially infectious materials that may result from the performance of an employee's duties.

Other Potentially Infectious Materials means (1) The following human body fluids: semen, vaginal secretions, cerebrospinal fluid, synovial fluid, pleural fluid, pericardial fluid, peritoneal fluid, amniotic fluid, saliva in dental procedures, any body fluid that is visibly contaminated with blood, and all body fluids in situations where it is difficult or impossible to differentiate between body fluids; (2) Any unfixed tissue or organ (other than intact skin) from a human (living or dead); and (3) HIV-containing cell or tissue cultures, organ cultures, and HIV- or HBV-containing culture medium or other solutions; and blood, organs, or other tissues from experimental animals infected with HIV or HBV.

Parenteral means piercing mucous membranes or the skin barrier through such events as needlesticks, human bites, cuts, and abrasions.

Personal Protective Equipment is specialized clothing or equipment worn by an employee for protection against a hazard. General work clothes (e.g., uniforms, pants, shirts or blouses) not intended to function as protection against a hazard are not considered to be personal protective equipment.

Production Facility means a facility engaged in industrial-scale, large-volume or high concentration production of HIV or HBV.

Regulated Waste means liquid or semi-liquid blood or other potentially infectious materials; contaminated items that would release blood or other potentially infectious materials in a liquid or semi-liquid state if compressed; items that are caked with dried blood or other potentially infectious materials and are capable of releasing these materials during handling; contaminated sharps; and pathological and microbiological wastes containing blood or other potentially infectious materials.

Research Laboratory means a laboratory producing or using research-laboratory-scale amounts of HIV or HBV. Research laboratories may produce high concentrations of HIV or HBV but not in the volume found in production facilities.

Sharps with Engineered Sharps Injury Protections means a nonneedle sharp or a needle device used for withdrawing body fluids, accessing a vein or artery, or administering medications or other fluids, with a built-in safety feature or mechanism that effectively reduces the risk of an exposure incident.

Source Individual means any individual, living or dead, whose blood or other potentially infectious materials may be a source of occupational exposure to the employee. Examples include, but are not limited to, hospital and clinic patients; clients in institutions for the developmentally disabled; trauma victims; clients of drug and alcohol treatment facilities; residents of hospices and nursing homes; human remains; and individuals who donate or sell blood or blood components.

Sterilize means the use of a physical or chemical procedure to destroy all microbial life including highly resistant bacterial endospores.

Universal Precautions is an approach to infection control. According to the concept of Universal Precautions, all human blood and certain human body fluids are treated as if known to be infectious for HIV, HBV, and other bloodborne pathogens.

Work Practice Controls means controls that reduce the likelihood of exposure by altering the manner in which a task is performed (e.g., prohibiting recapping of needles by a two-handed technique).

(c) **Exposure Control -**

(c)(1) **Exposure Control Plan.**

(c)(1)(i) Each employer having an employee(s) with occupational exposure as defined by paragraph (b) of this section shall establish a written Exposure Control Plan designed to eliminate or minimize employee exposure.

(c)(1)(ii) The Exposure Control Plan shall contain at least the following elements:

(c)(1)(ii)(A) The exposure determination required by paragraph (c)(2),

(c)(1)(ii)(B) The schedule and method of implementation for paragraphs (d) Methods of Compliance, (e) HIV and HBV Research Laboratories and Production Facilities, (f) Hepatitis B Vaccination and Post-Exposure Evaluation and Follow-up, (g) Communication of Hazards to Employees, and (h) Recordkeeping, of this standard, and

(c)(1)(ii)(C) The procedure for the evaluation of circumstances surrounding exposure incidents as required by paragraph (f)(3)(i) of this standard.

(c)(1)(iii) Each employer shall ensure that a copy of the Exposure Control Plan is accessible to employees in accordance with 29 CFR 1910.1020(e).

(c)(1)(iv) The Exposure Control Plan shall be reviewed and updated at least annually and whenever necessary to reflect new or modified tasks and procedures which affect occupational exposure and to reflect new or revised employee positions with occupational exposure. The review and update of such plans shall also:

(c)(1)(iv)(A) reflect changes in technology that eliminate or reduce exposure to bloodborne pathogens; and

(c)(1)(iv)(B) document annually consideration and implementation of appropriate commercially available and effective safer medical devices designed to eliminate or minimize occupational exposure.

(c)(1)(v) An employer, who is required to establish an Exposure Control Plan shall solicit input from non-managerial employees responsible for direct patient care who are potentially exposed to injuries from contaminated sharps in the identification, evaluation, and selection of effective engineering and work practice controls and shall document the solicitation in the Exposure Control Plan.

(c)(1)(vi) The Exposure Control Plan shall be made available to the Assistant Secretary and the Director upon request for examination and copying.

(c)(2) **Exposure Determination**.

(c)(2)(i) Each employer who has an employee(s) with occupational exposure as defined by paragraph (b) of this section shall prepare an exposure determination. This exposure determination shall contain the following:

(c)(2)(i)(A) A list of all job classifications in which all employees in those job classifications have occupational exposure;

(c)(2)(i)(B) A list of job classifications in which some employees have occupational exposure, and (c)(2)(i)(C) A list of all tasks and procedures or groups of closely related task and procedures in which occupational exposure occurs and that are performed by employees in job classifications listed in accordance with the provisions of paragraph (c)(2)(i)(B) of this standard.

(c)(2)(ii) This exposure determination shall be made without regard to the use of personal protective equipment.

(d) **Methods of Compliance -**

(d)(1) **General**. Universal precautions shall be observed to prevent contact with blood or other potentially infectious materials. Under circumstances in which differentiation between body fluid types is difficult or impossible, all body fluids shall be considered potentially infectious materials.

(d)(2) **Engineering and Work Practice Controls**.

(d)(2)(i) Engineering and work practice controls shall be used to eliminate or minimize employee exposure. Where occupational exposure remains after institution of these controls, personal protective equipment shall also be used.

(d)(2)(ii) Engineering controls shall be examined and maintained or replaced on a regular schedule to ensure their effectiveness.

(d)(2)(iii) Employers shall provide handwashing facilities which are readily accessible to employees.

(d)(2)(iv) When provision of handwashing facilities is not feasible, the employer shall provide either an appropriate antiseptic hand cleanser in conjunction with clean cloth/paper towels or antiseptic towelettes. When antiseptic hand cleansers or towelettes are used, hands shall be washed with soap and running water as soon as feasible.

(d)(2)(v) Employers shall ensure that employees wash their hands immediately or as soon as feasible after removal of gloves or other personal protective equipment.

(d)(2)(vi) Employers shall ensure that employees wash hands and any other skin with soap and water, or flush mucous membranes with water immediately or as soon as feasible following contact of such body areas with blood or other potentially infectious materials.

(d)(2)(vii) Contaminated needles and other contaminated sharps shall not be bent, recapped, or removed except as noted in paragraphs (d)(2)(vii)(A) and (d)(2)(vii)(B) below. Shearing or breaking of contaminated needles is prohibited.

(d)(2)(vii)(A) Contaminated needles and other contaminated sharps shall not be bent, recapped or removed unless the employer can demonstrate that no alternative is feasible or that such action is required by a specific medical or dental procedure.

(d)(2)(vii)(B) Such bending, recapping or needle removal must be accomplished through the use of a mechanical device or a one-handed technique.

(d)(2)(viii) Immediately or as soon as possible after use, contaminated reusable sharps shall be placed in appropriate containers until properly reprocessed. These containers shall be:

(d)(2)(viii)(A) puncture resistant;

(d)(2)(viii)(B) labeled or color-coded in accordance with this standard;

(d)(2)(viii)(C) leakproof on the sides and bottom; and

(d)(2)(viii)(D) in accordance with the requirements set forth in paragraph (d)(4)(ii)(E) for reusable sharps.

(d)(2)(ix) Eating, drinking, smoking, applying cosmetics or lip balm, and handling contact lenses are prohibited in work areas where there is a reasonable likelihood of occupational exposure.

(d)(2)(x) Food and drink shall not be kept in refrigerators, freezers, shelves, cabinets or on countertops or benchtops where blood or other potentially infectious materials are present.

(d)(2)(xi) All procedures involving blood or other potentially infectious materials shall be performed in such a manner as to minimize splashing, spraying, spattering, and generation of droplets of these substances.

(d)(2)(xii) Mouth pipetting/suctioning of blood or other potentially infectious materials is prohibited.

(d)(2)(xiii) Specimens of blood or other potentially infectious materials shall be placed in a container which prevents leakage during collection, handling, processing, storage, transport, or shipping.

(d)(2)(xiii)(A) The container for storage, transport, or shipping shall be labeled or color-coded according to paragraph (g)(1)(i) and closed prior to being stored, transported, or shipped. When a facility utilizes Universal Precautions in the handling of all specimens, the labeling/color-coding of specimens is not necessary provided containers are recognizable as containing specimens. This exemption only applies while such specimens/containers remain within the facility. Labeling or color-coding in accordance with paragraph (g)(1)(i) is required when such specimens/containers leave the facility.

(d)(2)(xiii)(B) If outside contamination of the primary container occurs, the primary container shall be placed within a second container which prevents leakage during handling, processing, storage, transport, or shipping and is labeled or color-coded according to the requirements of this standard.

(d)(2)(xiii)(C) If the specimen could puncture the primary container, the primary container shall be placed within a secondary container which is puncture-resistant in addition to the above characteristics.

(d)(2)(xiv) Equipment which may become contaminated with blood or other potentially infectious materials shall be examined prior to servicing or shipping and shall be decontaminated as necessary, unless the employer can demonstrate that decontamination of such equipment or portions of such equipment is not feasible.

(d)(2)(xiv)(A) A readily observable label in accordance with paragraph (g)(1)(i)(H) shall be attached to the equipment stating which portions remain contaminated.

(d)(2)(xiv)(B) The employer shall ensure that this information is conveyed to all affected employees, the servicing representative, and/or the manufacturer, as appropriate, prior to handling, servicing, or shipping so that appropriate precautions will be taken.

(d)(3) **Personal Protective Equipment -**

(d)(3)(i) **Provision**. When there is occupational exposure, the employer shall provide, at no cost to the employee, appropriate personal protective equipment such as, but not limited to, gloves, gowns, laboratory coats, face shields or masks and eye protection, and mouthpieces, resuscitation bags, pocket masks, or other ventilation devices. Personal protective equipment will be considered "appropriate" only if it does not permit blood or other potentially infectious materials to pass through to or reach the employee's work clothes, street clothes, undergarments, skin, eyes, mouth, or other mucous membranes under normal conditions of use and for the duration of time which the protective equipment will be used.

(d)(3)(ii) **Use**. The employer shall ensure that the employee uses appropriate personal protective equipment unless the employer shows that the employee temporarily and briefly declined to use personal protective equipment when, under rare and extraordinary circumstances, it was the employee's professional judgment that in the specific instance its use would have prevented the delivery of health care or public safety services or would have posed an increased hazard to the safety of the worker or co-worker. When the employee makes this judgement, the circumstances shall be investigated and documented in order to determine whether changes can be instituted to prevent such occurrences in the future.

(d)(3)(iii) **Accessibility**. The employer shall ensure that appropriate personal protective equipment in the appropriate sizes is readily accessible at the worksite or is issued to employees. Hypoallergenic gloves, glove liners, powderless gloves, or other similar alternatives shall be readily accessible to those employees who are allergic to the gloves normally provided.

(d)(3)(iv) **Cleaning, Laundering, and Disposal**. The employer shall clean, launder, and dispose of personal protective equipment required by paragraphs (d) and (e) of this standard, at no cost to the employee.

(d)(3)(v) **Repair and Replacement**. The employer shall repair or replace personal protective equipment as needed to maintain its effectiveness, at no cost to the employee.

(d)(3)(vi) If a garment(s) is penetrated by blood or other potentially infectious materials, the garment(s) shall be removed immediately or as soon as feasible.

(d)(3)(vii) All personal protective equipment shall be removed prior to leaving the work area.

(d)(3)(viii) When personal protective equipment is removed it shall be placed in an appropriately designated area or container for storage, washing, decontamination or disposal.

(d)(3)(ix) **Gloves**. Gloves shall be worn when it can be reasonably anticipated that the employee may have hand contact with blood, other potentially infectious materials, mucous membranes, and non-intact skin; when performing vascular access procedures except as specified in paragraph (d)(3)(ix)(D); and when handling or touching contaminated items or surfaces.

(d)(3)(ix)(A) Disposable (single use) gloves such as surgical or examination gloves, shall be replaced as soon as practical when contaminated or as soon as feasible if they are torn, punctured, or when their ability to function as a barrier is compromised.

(d)(3)(ix)(B) Disposable (single use) gloves shall not be washed or decontaminated for re-use.

(d)(3)(ix)(C) Utility gloves may be decontaminated for re-use if the integrity of the glove is not compromised. However, they must be discarded if they are cracked, peeling, torn, punctured, or exhibit other signs of deterioration or when their ability to function as a barrier is compromised.

(d)(3)(ix)(D) If an employer in a volunteer blood donation center judges that routine gloving for all phlebotomies is not necessary then the employer shall:

(d)(3)(ix)(D)(**1**) Periodically reevaluate this policy;

(d)(3)(ix)(D)(**2**) Make gloves available to all employees who wish to use them for phlebotomy;

(d)(3)(ix)(D)(**3**) Not discourage the use of gloves for phlebotomy; and

(d)(3)(ix)(D)(**4**) Require that gloves be used for phlebotomy in the following circumstances:

(d)(3)(ix)(D)(**4**)(**i**) When the employee has cuts, scratches, or other breaks in his or her skin;

(d)(3)(ix)(D)(**4**)(**ii**) When the employee judges that hand contamination with blood may occur, for example, when performing phlebotomy on an uncooperative source individual; and

(d)(3)(ix)(D)(**4**)(**iii**) When the employee is receiving training in phlebotomy.

(d)(3)(x) **Masks, Eye Protection, and Face Shields**. Masks in combination with eye protection devices, such as goggles or glasses with solid side shields, or chin-length face shields, shall be worn whenever splashes, spray, spatter, or droplets of blood or other potentially infectious materials may be generated and eye, nose, or mouth contamination can be reasonably anticipated.

(d)(3)(xi) **Gowns, Aprons, and Other Protective Body Clothing**. Appropriate protective clothing such as, but not limited to, gowns, aprons, lab coats, clinic jackets, or similar outer garments shall be worn in occupational exposure situations. The type and characteristics will depend upon the task and degree of exposure anticipated.

(d)(3)(xii) Surgical caps or hoods and/or shoe covers or boots shall be worn in instances when gross contamination can reasonably be anticipated (e.g., autopsies, orthopaedic surgery).

(d)(4) **Housekeeping -**

(d)(4)(i) **General**. Employers shall ensure that the worksite is maintained in a clean and sanitary condition. The employer shall determine and implement an appropriate written schedule for cleaning and method of decontamination based upon the location within the facility, type of surface to be cleaned, type of soil present, and tasks or procedures being performed in the area.

(d)(4)(ii) All equipment and environmental and working surfaces shall be cleaned and decontaminated after contact with blood or other potentially infectious materials.

(d)(4)(ii)(A) Contaminated work surfaces shall be decontaminated with an appropriate disinfectant after completion of procedures; immediately or as soon as feasible when surfaces are overtly contaminated or after any spill of blood or other potentially infectious materials; and at the end of the work shift if the surface may have become contaminated since the last cleaning.

(d)(4)(ii)(B) Protective coverings, such as plastic wrap, aluminum foil, or imperviously-backed absorbent paper used to cover equipment and environmental surfaces, shall be removed and replaced as soon as feasible when they become overtly contaminated or at the end of the workshift if they may have become contaminated during the shift.

(d)(4)(ii)(C) All bins, pails, cans, and similar receptacles intended for reuse which have a reasonable likelihood for becoming contaminated with blood or other potentially infectious materials shall be inspected and decontaminated on a regularly scheduled basis and cleaned and decontaminated immediately or as soon as feasible upon visible contamination.

(d)(4)(ii)(D) Broken glassware which may be contaminated shall not be picked up directly with the hands. It shall be cleaned up using mechanical means, such as a brush and dust pan, tongs, or forceps.

(d)(4)(ii)(E) Reusable sharps that are contaminated with blood or other potentially infectious materials shall not be stored or processed in a manner that requires employees to reach by hand into the containers where these sharps have been placed.

(d)(4)(iii) **Regulated Waste---**

(d)(4)(iii)(A) **Contaminated Sharps Discarding and Containment**.

(d)(4)(iii)(A)(**1**) Contaminated sharps shall be discarded immediately or as soon as feasible in containers that are:

(d)(4)(iii)(A)(**1**)(**i**) Closable;

(d)(4)(iii)(A)(**1**)(**ii**) Puncture resistant;

(d)(4)(iii)(A)(**1**)(**iii**) Leakproof on sides and bottom; and

(d)(4)(iii)(A)(**1**)(**iv**) Labeled or color-coded in accordance with paragraph (g)(1)(i) of this standard.

(d)(4)(iii)(A)(**2**) During use, containers for contaminated sharps shall be:

(d)(4)(iii)(A)(**2**)(**i**) Easily accessible to personnel and located as close as is feasible to the immediate area where sharps are used or can be reasonably anticipated to be found (e.g., laundries);

(d)(4)(iii)(A)(**2**)(**ii**) Maintained upright throughout use; and

(d)(4)(iii)(A)(**2**)(**iii**) Replaced routinely and not be allowed to overfill.

(d)(4)(iii)(A)(**3**) When moving containers of contaminated sharps from the area of use, the containers shall be:

(d)(4)(iii)(A)(**3**)(**i**) Closed immediately prior to removal or replacement to prevent spillage or protrusion of contents during handling, storage, transport, or shipping;

(d)(4)(iii)(A)(**3**)(**ii**) Placed in a secondary container if leakage is possible. The second container shall be:

(d)(4)(iii)(A)(**3**)(**ii**)(**A**) Closable;

(d)(4)(iii)(A)(**3**)(**ii**)(**B**) Constructed to contain all contents and prevent leakage during handling, storage, transport, or shipping; and

(d)(4)(iii)(A)(**3**)(**ii**)(**C**) Labeled or color-coded according to paragraph (g)(1)(i) of this standard.

(d)(4)(iii)(A)(**4**) Reusable containers shall not be opened, emptied, or cleaned manually or in any other manner which would expose employees to the risk of percutaneous injury.

(d)(4)(iii)(B) **Other Regulated Waste Containment -**

(d)(4)(iii)(B)(1) Regulated waste shall be placed in containers which are:

(d)(4)(iii)(B)(1)(**i**) Closable;

(d)(4)(iii)(B)(1)(**ii**) Constructed to contain all contents and prevent leakage of fluids during handling, storage, transport or shipping;

(d)(4)(iii)(B)(1)(**iii**) Labeled or color-coded in accordance with paragraph (g)(1)(i) this standard; and

(d)(4)(iii)(B)(1)(**iv**) Closed prior to removal to prevent spillage or protrusion of contents during handling, storage, transport, or shipping.

(d)(4)(iii)(B)(**2**) If outside contamination of the regulated waste container occurs, it shall be placed in a second container. The second container shall be:

(d)(4)(iii)(B)(**2**)(**i**) Closable;

(d)(4)(iii)(B)(**2**)(**ii**) Constructed to contain all contents and prevent leakage of fluids during handling, storage, transport or shipping;

(d)(4)(iii)(B)(**2**)(**iii**) Labeled or color-coded in accordance with paragraph (g)(1)(i) of this standard; and (d)(4)(iii)(B)(**2**)(**iv**) Closed prior to removal to prevent spillage or protrusion of contents during handling, storage, transport, or shipping.

(d)(4)(iii)(C) Disposal of all regulated waste shall be in accordance with applicable regulations of the United States, States and Territories, and political subdivisions of States and Territories.

(d)(4)(iv) **Laundry**.

(d)(4)(iv)(A) Contaminated laundry shall be handled as little as possible with a minimum of agitation.

(d)(4)(iv)(A)(1) Contaminated laundry shall be bagged or containerized at the location where it was used and shall not be sorted or rinsed in the location of use.

(d)(4)(iv)(A)(2) Contaminated laundry shall be placed and transported in bags or containers labeled or color-coded in accordance with paragraph (g)(1)(i) of this standard. When a facility utilizes Universal Precautions in the handling of all soiled laundry, alternative labeling or color-coding is sufficient if it permits all employees to recognize the containers as requiring compliance with Universal Precautions.

(d)(4)(iv)(A)(3) Whenever contaminated laundry is wet and presents a reasonable likelihood of soak-through of or leakage from the bag or container, the laundry shall be placed and transported in bags or containers which prevent soak-through and/or leakage of fluids to the exterior.

(d)(4)(iv)(B) The employer shall ensure that employees who have contact with contaminated laundry wear protective gloves and other appropriate personal protective equipment.

(d)(4)(iv)(C) When a facility ships contaminated laundry off-site to a second facility which does not utilize Universal Precautions in the handling of all laundry, the facility generating the contaminated laundry must place such laundry in bags or containers which are labeled or color-coded in accordance with paragraph (g)(1)(i).

(e) **HIV and HBV Research Laboratories and Production Facilities**.

(e)(1) This paragraph applies to research laboratories and production facilities engaged in the culture, production, concentration, experimentation, and manipulation of HIV and HBV. It does not apply to clinical or diagnostic laboratories engaged solely in the analysis of blood, tissues, or organs. These requirements apply in addition to the other requirements of the standard.

(e)(2) Research laboratories and production facilities shall meet the following criteria:

(e)(2)(i) **Standard Microbiological Practices**. All regulated waste shall either be incinerated or decontaminated by a method such as autoclaving known to effectively destroy bloodborne pathogens.

(e)(2)(ii) **Special Practices**.

(e)(2)(ii)(A) Laboratory doors shall be kept closed when work involving HIV or HBV is in progress.

(e)(2)(ii)(B) Contaminated materials that are to be decontaminated at a site away from the work area shall be placed in a durable, leakproof, labeled or color-coded container that is closed before being removed from the work area.

(e)(2)(ii)(C) Access to the work area shall be limited to authorized persons. Written policies and procedures shall be established whereby only persons who have been advised of the potential biohazard, who meet any specific entry requirements, and who comply with all entry and exit procedures shall be allowed to enter the work areas and animal rooms.

(e)(2)(ii)(D) When other potentially infectious materials or infected animals are present in the work area or containment module, a hazard warning sign incorporating the universal biohazard symbol shall be posted on all access doors. The hazard warning sign shall comply with paragraph (g)(1)(ii) of this standard.

(e)(2)(ii)(E) All activities involving other potentially infectious materials shall be conducted in biological safety cabinets or other physical-containment devices within the containment module. No work with these other potentially infectious materials shall be conducted on the open bench.

(e)(2)(ii)(F) Laboratory coats, gowns, smocks, uniforms, or other appropriate protective clothing shall be used in the work area and animal rooms. Protective clothing shall not be worn outside of the work area and shall be decontaminated before being laundered.

(e)(2)(ii)(G) Special care shall be taken to avoid skin contact with other potentially infectious materials. Gloves shall be worn when handling infected animals and when making hand contact with other potentially infectious materials is unavoidable.

(e)(2)(ii)(H) Before disposal all waste from work areas and from animal rooms shall either be incinerated or decontaminated by a method such as autoclaving known to effectively destroy bloodborne pathogens.

(e)(2)(ii)(I) Vacuum lines shall be protected with liquid disinfectant traps and high-efficiency particulate air (HEPA) filters or filters of equivalent or superior efficiency and which are checked routinely and maintained or replaced as necessary.

(e)(2)(ii)(J) Hypodermic needles and syringes shall be used only for parenteral injection and aspiration of fluids from laboratory animals and diaphragm bottles. Only needle-locking syringes or disposable syringe-needle units (i.e., the needle is integral to the syringe) shall be used for the injection or aspiration of other potentially infectious materials. Extreme caution shall be used when handling needles and syringes. A needle shall not be bent, sheared, replaced in the sheath or guard, or removed from the syringe following use. The needle and syringe shall be promptly placed in a puncture-resistant container and autoclaved or decontaminated before reuse or disposal.

(e)(2)(ii)(K) All spills shall be immediately contained and cleaned up by appropriate professional staff or others properly trained and equipped to work with potentially concentrated infectious materials.

(e)(2)(ii)(L) A spill or accident that results in an exposure incident shall be immediately reported to the laboratory director or other responsible person.

(e)(2)(ii)(M) A biosafety manual shall be prepared or adopted and periodically reviewed and updated at least annually or more often if necessary. Personnel shall be advised of potential hazards, shall be required to read instructions on practices and procedures, and shall be required to follow them.

(e)(2)(iii) **Containment Equipment**.

(e)(2)(iii)(A) Certified biological safety cabinets (Class I, II, or III) or other appropriate combinations of personal protection or physical containment devices, such as special protective clothing, respirators, centrifuge safety cups, sealed centrifuge rotors, and containment caging for animals, shall be used for all activities with other potentially infectious materials that pose a threat of exposure to droplets, splashes, spills, or aerosols.

(e)(2)(iii)(B) Biological safety cabinets shall be certified when installed, whenever they are moved and at least annually.

(e)(3) HIV and HBV research laboratories shall meet the following criteria:

(e)(3)(i) Each laboratory shall contain a facility for hand washing and an eye wash facility which is readily available within the work area.

(e)(3)(ii) An autoclave for decontamination of regulated waste shall be available.

(e)(4) HIV and HBV production facilities shall meet the following criteria:

(e)(4)(i) The work areas shall be separated from areas that are open to unrestricted traffic flow within the building. Passage through two sets of doors shall be the basic requirement for entry into the work area from access corridors or other contiguous areas. Physical separation of the high-containment work area from access corridors or other areas or activities may also be provided by a double-doored clothes-change room (showers may be included), airlock, or other access facility that requires passing through two sets of doors before entering the work area.

(e)(4)(ii) The surfaces of doors, walls, floors and ceilings in the work area shall be water resistant so that they can be easily cleaned. Penetrations in these surfaces shall be sealed or capable of being sealed to facilitate decontamination.

(e)(4)(iii) Each work area shall contain a sink for washing hands and a readily available eye wash facility. The sink shall be foot, elbow, or automatically operated and shall be located near the exit door of the work area.

(e)(4)(iv) Access doors to the work area or containment module shall be self-closing.

(e)(4)(v) An autoclave for decontamination of regulated waste shall be available within or as near as possible to the work area.

(e)(4)(vi) A ducted exhaust-air ventilation system shall be provided. This system shall create directional airflow that draws air into the work area through the entry area. The exhaust air shall not be recirculated to any other area of the building, shall be discharged to the outside, and shall be dispersed away from occupied areas and air intakes. The proper direction of the airflow shall be verified (i.e., into the work area).

(e)(5) **Training Requirements**. Additional training requirements for employees in HIV and HBV research laboratories and HIV and HBV production facilities are specified in paragraph (g)(2)(ix).

(f) **Hepatitis B Vaccination and Post-exposure Evaluation and Follow-up -**

(f)(1) **General**.

(f)(1)(i) The employer shall make available the hepatitis B vaccine and vaccination series to all employees who have occupational exposure, and post-exposure evaluation and follow-up to all employees who have had an exposure incident.

(f)(1)(ii) The employer shall ensure that all medical evaluations and procedures including the hepatitis B vaccine and vaccination series and post-exposure evaluation and follow-up, including prophylaxis, are:

(f)(1)(ii)(A) Made available at no cost to the employee;

(f)(1)(ii)(B) Made available to the employee at a reasonable time and place;

(f)(1)(ii)(C) Performed by or under the supervision of a licensed physician or by or under the supervision of another licensed healthcare professional; and (f)(1)(ii)(D) Provided according to recommendations of the U.S. Public Health Service current at the time these evaluations and procedures take place, except as specified by this paragraph (f).

(f)(1)(iii) The employer shall ensure that all laboratory tests are conducted by an accredited laboratory at no cost to the employee.

(f)(2) **Hepatitis B Vaccination**.

(f)(2)(i) Hepatitis B vaccination shall be made available after the employee has received the training required in paragraph (g)(2)(vii)(I) and within 10 working days of initial assignment to all employees who have occupational exposure unless the employee has previously received the complete hepatitis B vaccination series, antibody testing has revealed that the employee is immune, or the vaccine is contraindicated for medical reasons.

(f)(2)(ii) The employer shall not make participation in a prescreening program a prerequisite for receiving hepatitis B vaccination.

(f)(2)(iii) If the employee initially declines hepatitis B vaccination but at a later date while still covered under the standard decides to accept the vaccination, the employer shall make available hepatitis B vaccination at that time.

(f)(2)(iv) The employer shall assure that employees who decline to accept hepatitis B vaccination offered by the employer sign the statement in Appendix A.

(f)(2)(v) If a routine booster dose(s) of hepatitis B vaccine is recommended by the U.S. Public Health Service at a future date, such booster dose(s) shall be made available in accordance with section (f)(1)(ii).

(f)(3) **Post-exposure Evaluation and Follow-up**. Following a report of an exposure incident, the employer shall make immediately available to the exposed employee a confidential medical evaluation and follow-up, including at least the following elements:

(f)(3)(i) Documentation of the route(s) of exposure, and the circumstances under which the exposure incident occurred;

(f)(3)(ii) Identification and documentation of the source individual, unless the employer can establish that identification is infeasible or prohibited by state or local law;

(f)(3)(ii)(A) The source individual's blood shall be tested as soon as feasible and after consent is obtained in order to determine HBV and HIV infectivity. If consent is not obtained, the employer shall establish that legally required consent cannot be obtained. When the source individual's consent is not required by law, the source individual's blood, if available, shall be tested and the results documented.

(f)(3)(ii)(B) When the source individual is already known to be infected with HBV or HIV, testing for the source individual's known HBV or HIV status need not be repeated.

(f)(3)(ii)(C) Results of the source individual's testing shall be made available to the exposed employee, and the employee shall be informed of applicable laws and regulations concerning disclosure of the identity and infectious status of the source individual.

(f)(3)(iii) Collection and testing of blood for HBV and HIV serological status;

(f)(3)(iii)(A) The exposed employee's blood shall be collected as soon as feasible and tested after consent is obtained.

(f)(3)(iii)(B) If the employee consents to baseline blood collection, but does not give consent at that time for HIV serologic testing, the sample shall be preserved for at least 90 days. If, within 90 days of the exposure incident, the employee elects to have the baseline sample tested, such testing shall be done as soon as feasible.

(f)(3)(iv) Post-exposure prophylaxis, when medically indicated, as recommended by the U.S. Public Health Service;

(f)(3)(v) Counseling; and

(f)(3)(vi) Evaluation of reported illnesses.

(f)(4) **Information Provided to the Healthcare Professional**.

(f)(4)(i) The employer shall ensure that the healthcare professional responsible for the employee's Hepatitis B vaccination is provided a copy of this regulation.

(f)(4)(ii) The employer shall ensure that the healthcare professional evaluating an employee after an exposure incident is provided the following information:

(f)(4)(ii)(A) A copy of this regulation;

(f)(4)(ii)(B) A description of the exposed employee's duties as they relate to the exposure incident;

(f)(4)(ii)(C) Documentation of the route(s) of exposure and circumstances under which exposure occurred;

(f)(4)(ii)(D) Results of the source individual's blood testing, if available; and

(f)(4)(ii)(E) All medical records relevant to the appropriate treatment of the employee including vaccination status which are the employer's responsibility to maintain.

(f)(5) **Healthcare Professional's Written Opinion**. The employer shall obtain and provide the employee with a copy of the evaluating healthcare professional's written opinion within 15 days of the completion of the evaluation.

(f)(5)(i) The healthcare professional's written opinion for Hepatitis B vaccination shall be limited to whether Hepatitis B vaccination is indicated for an employee, and if the employee has received such vaccination.

(f)(5)(ii) The healthcare professional's written opinion for post-exposure evaluation and follow-up shall be limited to the following information:

(f)(5)(ii)(A) That the employee has been informed of the results of the evaluation; and

(f)(5)(ii)(B) That the employee has been told about any medical conditions resulting from exposure to blood or other potentially infectious materials which require further evaluation or treatment.

(f)(5)(iii) All other findings or diagnoses shall remain confidential and shall not be included in the written report.

(f)(6) **Medical Recordkeeping**. Medical records required by this standard shall be maintained in accordance with paragraph (h)(1) of this section.

(g) **Communication of Hazards to Employees -**

(g)(1) **Labels and Signs -**

(g)(1)(i) **Labels**.

(g)(1)(i)(A) Warning labels shall be affixed to containers of regulated waste, refrigerators and freezers containing blood or other potentially infectious material; and other containers used to store, transport or ship blood or other potentially infectious materials, except as provided in paragraph (g)(1)(i)(E), (F) and (G).

(g)(1)(i)(B) Labels required by this section shall include the following legend:

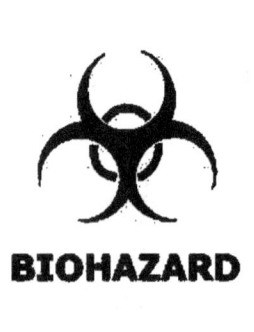

BIOHAZARD

(g)(1)(i)(C) These labels shall be fluorescent orange or orange-red or predominantly so, with lettering and symbols in a contrasting color.

(g)(1)(i)(D) Labels shall be affixed as close as feasible to the container by string, wire, adhesive, or other method that prevents their loss or unintentional removal.

(g)(1)(i)(E) Red bags or red containers may be substituted for labels.

(g)(1)(i)(F) Containers of blood, blood components, or blood products that are labeled as to their contents and have been released for transfusion or other clinical use are exempted from the labeling requirements of paragraph (g).

(g)(1)(i)(G) Individual containers of blood or other potentially infectious materials that are placed in a labeled container during storage, transport, shipment or disposal are exempted from the labeling requirement.

(g)(1)(i)(H) Labels required for contaminated equipment shall be in accordance with this paragraph and shall also state which portions of the equipment remain contaminated.

(g)(1)(i)(I) Regulated waste that has been decontaminated need not be labeled or color-coded.

(g)(1)(ii) **Signs**.

(g)(1)(ii)(A) The employer shall post signs at the entrance to work areas specified in paragraph (e), HIV and HBV Research Laboratory and Production Facilities, which shall bear the following legend:

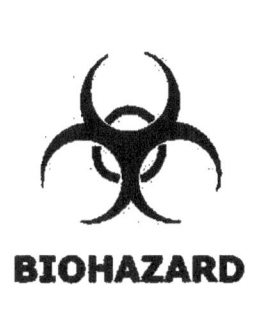

BIOHAZARD

(Name of the Infectious Agent)
(Special requirements for entering the area)
(Name, telephone number of the laboratory director or other responsible person.)

(g)(1)(ii)(B) These signs shall be fluorescent orange-red or predominantly so, with lettering and symbols in a contrasting color.

(g)(2) **Information and Training**.

(g)(2)(i) Employers shall ensure that all employees with occupational exposure participate in a training program which must be provided at no cost to the employee and during working hours.

(g)(2)(ii) Training shall be provided as follows:

(g)(2)(ii)(A) At the time of initial assignment to tasks where occupational exposure may take place;

(g)(2)(ii)(B) Within 90 days after the effective date of the standard; and

(g)(2)(ii)(C) At least annually thereafter.

(g)(2)(iii) For employees who have received training on bloodborne pathogens in the year preceding the effective date of the standard, only training with respect to the provisions of the standard which were not included need be provided.

(g)(2)(iv) Annual training for all employees shall be provided within one year of their previous training.

(g)(2)(v) Employers shall provide additional training when changes such as modification of tasks or procedures or institution of new tasks or procedures affect the employee's occupational exposure. The additional training may be limited to addressing the new exposures created.

(g)(2)(vi) Material appropriate in content and vocabulary to educational level, literacy, and language of employees shall be used.

(g)(2)(vii) The training program shall contain at a minimum the following elements:

(g)(2)(vii)(A) An accessible copy of the regulatory text of this standard and an explanation of its contents;

(g)(2)(vii)(B) A general explanation of the epidemiology and symptoms of bloodborne diseases;

(g)(2)(vii)(C) An explanation of the modes of transmission of bloodborne pathogens;

(g)(2)(vii)(D) An explanation of the employer's exposure control plan and the means by which the employee can obtain a copy of the written plan;

(g)(2)(vii)(E) An explanation of the appropriate methods for recognizing tasks and other activities that may involve exposure to blood and other potentially infectious materials;

(g)(2)(vii)(F) An explanation of the use and limitations of methods that will prevent or reduce exposure including appropriate engineering controls, work practices, and personal protective equipment;

(g)(2)(vii)(G) Information on the types, proper use, location, removal, handling, decontamination and disposal of personal protective equipment;

(g)(2)(vii)(H) An explanation of the basis for selection of personal protective equipment;

(g)(2)(vii)(I) Information on the hepatitis B vaccine, including information on its efficacy, safety, method of administration, the benefits of being vaccinated, and that the vaccine and vaccination will be offered free of charge;

(g)(2)(vii)(J) Information on the appropriate actions to take and persons to contact in an emergency involving blood or other potentially infectious materials;

(g)(2)(vii)(K) An explanation of the procedure to follow if an exposure incident occurs, including the method of reporting the incident and the medical follow-up that will be made available;

(g)(2)(vii)(L) Information on the post-exposure evaluation and follow-up that the employer is required to provide for the employee following an exposure incident;

(g)(2)(vii)(M) An explanation of the signs and labels and/or color coding required by paragraph (g)(1); and

(g)(2)(vii)(N) An opportunity for interactive questions and answers with the person conducting the training session.

(g)(2)(viii) The person conducting the training shall be knowledgeable in the subject matter covered by the elements contained in the training program as it relates to the workplace that the training will address.

(g)(2)(ix) Additional Initial Training for Employees in HIV and HBV Laboratories and Production Facilities. Employees in HIV or HBV research laboratories and HIV or HBV production facilities shall receive the following initial training in addition to the above training requirements.

(g)(2)(ix)(A) The employer shall assure that employees demonstrate proficiency in standard microbiological practices and techniques and in the practices and operations specific to the facility before being allowed to work with HIV or HBV.

(g)(2)(ix)(B) The employer shall assure that employees have prior experience in the handling of human pathogens or tissue cultures before working with HIV or HBV.

(g)(2)(ix)(C) The employer shall provide a training program to employees who have no prior experience in handling human pathogens. Initial work activities shall not include the handling of infectious agents. A progression of work activities shall be assigned as techniques are learned and proficiency is developed. The employer shall assure that employees participate in work activities involving infectious agents only after proficiency has been demonstrated.

(h) **Recordkeeping -**

(h)(1) **Medical Records.**

(h)(1)(i) The employer shall establish and maintain an accurate record for each employee with occupational exposure, in accordance with 29 CFR 1910.1020.

(h)(1)(ii) This record shall include:

(h)(1)(ii)(A) The name and social security number of the employee;

(h)(1)(ii)(B) A copy of the employee's hepatitis B vaccination status including the dates of all the hepatitis B vaccinations and any medical records relative to the employee's ability to receive vaccination as required by paragraph (f)(2);

(h)(1)(ii)(C) A copy of all results of examinations, medical testing, and follow-up procedures as required by paragraph (f)(3);

(h)(1)(ii)(D) The employer's copy of the healthcare professional's written opinion as required by paragraph (f)(5); and

(h)(1)(ii)(E) A copy of the information provided to the healthcare professional as required by paragraphs (f)(4)(ii)(B)(C) and (D).

(h)(1)(iii) Confidentiality. The employer shall ensure that employee medical records required by paragraph (h)(1) are:

(h)(1)(iii)(A) Kept confidential; and

(h)(1)(iii)(B) Not disclosed or reported without the employee's express written consent to any person within or outside the workplace except as required by this section or as may be required by law.

(h)(1)(iv) The employer shall maintain the records required by paragraph (h) for at least the duration of employment plus 30 years in accordance with 29 CFR 1910.1020.

(h)(2) **Training Records.**

(h)(2)(i) Training records shall include the following information:

(h)(2)(i)(A) The dates of the training sessions;

(h)(2)(i)(B) The contents or a summary of the training sessions;

(h)(2)(i)(C) The names and qualifications of persons conducting the training; and

(h)(2)(i)(D) The names and job titles of all persons attending the training sessions.

(h)(2)(ii) Training records shall be maintained for 3 years from the date on which the training occurred.

(h)(3) **Availability**.

(h)(3)(i) The employer shall ensure that all records required to be maintained by this section shall be made available upon request to the Assistant Secretary and the Director for examination and copying.

(h)(3)(ii) Employee training records required by this paragraph shall be provided upon request for examination and copying to employees, to employee representatives, to the Director, and to the Assistant Secretary.

(h)(3)(iii) Employee medical records required by this paragraph shall be provided upon request for examination and copying to the subject employee, to anyone having written consent of the subject employee, to the Director, and to the Assistant Secretary in accordance with 29 CFR 1910.1020.

(h)(4) **Transfer of Records**.

(h)(4)(i) The employer shall comply with the requirements involving transfer of records set forth in 29 CFR 1910.1020(h).

(h)(4)(ii) If the employer ceases to do business and there is no successor employer to receive and retain the records for the prescribed period, the employer shall notify the Director, at least three months prior to their disposal and transmit them to the Director, if required by the Director to do so, within that three month period.

(h)(5) **Sharps Injury Log**.

(h)(5)(i) The employer shall establish and maintain a sharps injury log for the recording of percutaneous injuries from contaminated sharps. The information in the sharps injury log shall be recorded and maintained in such manner as to protect the confidentiality of the injured employee. The sharps injury log shall contain, at a minimum:

(h)(5)(i)(A) the type and brand of device involved in the incident,

(h)(5)(i)(B) the department or work area where the exposure incident occurred, and (h)(5)(i)(C) an explanation of how the incident occurred.

(h)(5)(ii) The requirement to establish and maintain a sharps injury log shall apply to any employer who is required to maintain a log of occupational injuries and illnesses under 29 CFR 1904.

(h)(5)(iii) The sharps injury log shall be maintained for the period required by 29 CFR 1904.6.

(i) **Dates -**

(i)(1) **Effective Date**. The standard shall become effective on March 6, 1992.

(i)(2) The Exposure Control Plan required by paragraph (c) of this section shall be completed on or before May 5, 1992.

(i)(3) Paragraph (g)(2) Information and Training and (h) Recordkeeping shall take effect on or before June 4, 1992.

(i)(4) Paragraphs (d)(2) Engineering and Work Practice Controls, (d)(3) Personal Protective Equipment, (d)(4) Housekeeping, (e) HIV and HBV Research Laboratories and Production Facilities, (f) Hepatitis B Vaccination and Post-Exposure Evaluation and Follow-up, and (g)(1) Labels and Signs, shall take effect July 6, 1992.

APPENDIX A TO SECTION 1910.1030 - HEPATITIS B DECLINATION (MANDATORY)

I understand that due to my occupational exposure to blood or other potentially infectious materials I may be at risk of acquiring hepatitis B virus (HBV) infection. I have been given the opportunity to be vaccinated with hepatitis B vaccine, at no charge to myself. However, I decline hepatitis B vaccination at this time. I understand that by declining this vaccine, I continue to be at risk of acquiring hepatitis B, a serious disease. If in the future I continue to have occupational exposure to blood or other potentially infectious materials and I want to be vaccinated with hepatitis B vaccine, I can receive the vaccination series at no charge to me.

APPENDIX B-4

Updated U.S. Public Health Service Guidelines for the Management of Occupational Exposures to HBV, HCV, and HIV and Recommendations for Postexposure Prophylaxis (*Morbidity and Mortality Weekly,* June 29, 2001 / 50(RR11);1-42)

Summary

This report updates and consolidates all previous U.S. Public Health Service recommendations for the management of health-care personnel (HCP) who have occupational exposure to blood and other body fluids that might contain hepatitis B virus (HBV), hepatitis C virus (HCV), or human immunodeficiency virus (HIV).

Recommendations for HBV postexposure management include initiation of the hepatitis B vaccine series to any susceptible, unvaccinated person who sustains an occupational blood or body fluid exposure. Postexposure prophylaxis (PEP) with hepatitis B immune globulin (HBIG) and/or hepatitis B vaccine series should be considered for occupational exposures after evaluation of the hepatitis B surface antigen status of the source and the vaccination and vaccine-response status of the exposed person. Guidance is provided to clinicians and exposed HCP for selecting the appropriate HBV PEP.

Immune globulin and antiviral agents (e.g., interferon with or without ribavirin) are not recommended for PEP of hepatitis C. For HCV postexposure management, the HCV status of the source and the exposed person should be determined, and for HCP exposed to an HCV positive source, follow-up HCV testing should be performed to determine if infection develops.

Recommendations for HIV PEP include a basic 4-week regimen of two drugs (zidovudine [ZDV] and lamivudine [3TC]; 3TC and stavudine [d4T]; or didanosine [ddI] and d4T) for most HIV exposures and an expanded regimen that includes the addition of a third drug for HIV exposures that pose an increased risk for transmission. When the source person's virus is known or suspected to be resistant to one or more of the drugs considered for the PEP regimen, the selection of drugs to which the source person's virus is unlikely to be resistant is recommended.

In addition, this report outlines several special circumstances (e.g., delayed exposure report, unknown source person, pregnancy in the exposed person, resistance of the source virus to antiretroviral agents, or toxicity of the PEP regimen) when consultation with local experts and/or the National Clinicians' Post-Exposure Prophylaxis Hotline ([PEPline] 1-888-448-4911) is advised.

Occupational exposures should be considered urgent medical concerns to ensure timely postexposure management and administration of HBIG, hepatitis B vaccine, and/or HIV PEP.

INTRODUCTION

Avoiding occupational blood exposures is the primary way to prevent transmission of hepatitis B virus (HBV), hepatitis C virus (HCV), and human immunodeficiency virus (HIV) in health-care settings (1). However, hepatitis B immunization and postexposure management are integral components of a complete program to prevent infection following bloodborne pathogen exposure and are important elements of workplace safety (2).

The U.S. Public Health Service (PHS) has published previous guidelines for the management of HIV exposures that included considerations for postexposure prophylaxis (PEP) (3--5). Since publication of the 1998 HIV exposure guidelines (5), several new antiretroviral agents have been approved by the Food and Drug Administration (FDA), and more information is available about the use and safety of HIV PEP (6--11). In addition, questions exist regarding considerations about PEP regimens when the source person's virus is known or suspected to be resistant to one or more of the antiretroviral agents that might be used for PEP. Concern also has arisen about the use of PEP when it is not warranted. Data indicate that some health-care personnel (HCP) take a full course of HIV PEP after exposures that do not confer an HIV transmission risk (10,11).

In September 1999, a meeting of a PHS interagency working group* and expert consultants was convened by CDC. The PHS working group decided to issue updated recommendations for the management of occupational exposure to HIV. In addition, the report was to include recommendations for the management of occupational HBV and HCV exposures so that a single document could comprehensively address the management of occupational exposures to bloodborne pathogens. This report updates and consolidates the previous PHS guidelines and recommendations for occupational HBV, HCV, and HIV exposure management for HCP. Specific practice recommendations for the management of occupational bloodborne pathogen exposures are outlined to assist health-care institutions with the implementation of these PHS guidelines (Appendices A and B). As relevant information becomes available, updates of these recommendations will be published. Recommendations for nonoccupational (e.g., sexual, pediatric, and perinatal) HBV, HCV, and HIV exposures are not addressed in these guidelines and can be found elsewhere (12--15).

Definition of Health-Care Personnel and Exposure

In this report, health-care personnel (HCP) are defined as persons (e.g., employees, students, contractors, attending clinicians, public-safety workers, or volunteers) whose activities involve contact with patients or with blood or other body fluids from patients in a health-care, laboratory, or public-safety setting. The potential exists for blood and body fluid exposure to other workers, and the same principles of exposure management could be applied to other settings.

An exposure that might place HCP at risk for HBV, HCV, or HIV infection is defined as a percutaneous injury (e.g., a needlestick or cut with a sharp object) or contact of mucous membrane or nonintact skin (e.g., exposed skin that is chapped, abraded, or afflicted with dermatitis) with blood, tissue, or other body fluids that are potentially infectious (*16,17*).

In addition to blood and body fluids containing visible blood, semen and vaginal secretions also are considered potentially infectious. Although semen and vaginal secretions have been implicated in the sexual transmission of HBV, HCV, and HIV, they have not been implicated in occupational transmission from patients to HCP. The following fluids also are considered potentially infectious: cerebrospinal fluid, synovial fluid, pleural fluid, peritoneal fluid, pericardial fluid, and amniotic fluid. The risk for transmission of HBV, HCV, and HIV infection from these fluids is unknown; the potential risk to HCP from occupational exposures has not been assessed by epidemiologic studies in health-care settings. Feces, nasal secretions, saliva, sputum, sweat, tears, urine, and vomitus are not considered potentially infectious unless they contain blood. The risk for transmission of HBV, HCV, and HIV infection from these fluids and materials is extremely low.

Any direct contact (i.e., contact without barrier protection) to concentrated virus in a research laboratory or production facility is considered an exposure that requires clinical evaluation. For human bites, the clinical evaluation must include the possibility that both the person bitten and the person who inflicted the bite were exposed to bloodborne pathogens. Transmission of HBV or HIV infection only rarely has been reported by this route (*18--20*) (CDC, unpublished data, 1998).

BACKGROUND

This section provides the rationale for the postexposure management and prophylaxis recommendations presented in this report. Additional details concerning the risk for occupational bloodborne pathogen transmission to HCP and management of occupational bloodborne pathogen exposures are available elsewhere (*5,12,13,21-24*).

Occupational Transmission of HBV

Risk for Occupational Transmission of HBV

HBV infection is a well recognized occupational risk for HCP (*25*). The risk of HBV infection is primarily related to the degree of contact with blood in the work place and also to the hepatitis B e antigen (HBeAg) status of the source person. In studies of HCP who sustained injuries from needles contaminated with blood containing HBV, the risk of developing clinical hepatitis if the blood was both hepatitis B surface antigen (HBsAg)- and HBeAg-positive was 22%--31%; the risk of developing serologic evidence of HBV infection was 37%--62%. By comparison, the risk of developing clinical hepatitis from a needle contaminated with HBsAg-positive, HBeAg-negative blood was 1%--6%, and the risk of developing serologic evidence of HBV infection, 23%--37% (*26*).

Although percutaneous injuries are among the most efficient modes of HBV transmission, these exposures probably account for only a minority of HBV infections among HCP. In several investigations of nosocomial hepatitis B outbreaks, most infected HCP could not recall an overt percutaneous injury (*27,28*), although in some studies, up to one third of infected HCP recalled caring for a patient who was HBsAg-positive (*29,30*). In addition, HBV has been demonstrated to survive in dried blood at room temperature on environmental surfaces for at least 1 week (*31*). Thus, HBV infections that occur in HCP with no history of nonoccupational exposure or occupational percutaneous injury might have resulted from direct or indirect blood or body fluid exposures that inoculated HBV into cutaneous scratches, abrasions, burns, other lesions, or on mucosal surfaces (*32--34*). The potential for HBV transmission through contact with environmental surfaces has been demonstrated in investigations of HBV outbreaks among patients and staff of hemodialysis units (*35--37*).

Blood contains the highest HBV titers of all body fluids and is the most important vehicle of transmission in the health-care setting. HBsAg is also found in several other body fluids, including breast milk, bile, cerebrospinal fluid, feces, nasopharyngeal washings, saliva, semen, sweat, and synovial fluid (*38*). However, the concentration of HBsAg in body fluids can be 100--1000---fold higher than the concentration of infectious HBV particles. Therefore, most body fluids are not efficient vehicles of transmission because they contain low quantities of infectious HBV, despite the presence of HBsAg.

In serologic studies conducted in the United States during the 1970s, HCP had a prevalence of HBV infection approximately 10 times higher than the general population (*39--42*). Because of the high risk of HBV infection among HCP, routine preexposure vaccination of HCP against hepatitis B and the use of standard precautions to prevent exposure to blood and other potentially infectious body fluids have been recommended since the early 1980s (*43*). Regulations issued by the Occupational Safety and Health Administration (OSHA) (*2*) have increased compliance with these recommendations. Since the implementation of these recommendations, a sharp decline has occurred in the incidence of HBV infection among HCP.

PEP for HBV

Efficacy of PEP for HBV. The effectiveness of hepatitis B immune globulin (HBIG) and/or hepatitis B vaccine in various postexposure settings has been evaluated by prospective studies. For perinatal exposure to an HBsAg-, HBeAg-positive mother, a regimen combining HBIG and initiation of the hepatitis B vaccine series at birth is 85%--95% effective in preventing HBV infection (*44,45*). Regimens involving either multiple doses of HBIG alone or the hepatitis B vaccine series alone are 70%--75% effective in preventing HBV infection (*46*). In the occupational setting, multiple doses of HBIG initiated within 1 week following percutaneous exposure to HBsAg-positive blood provides an estimated 75% protection from HBV infection (*47--49*). Although the postexposure efficacy of the combination of HBIG and the hepatitis B vaccine series has not been evaluated in the occupational setting, the increased efficacy of this regimen observed in the perinatal setting, compared with HBIG alone, is presumed to apply to the occupational setting as well. In addition, because persons requiring PEP in the occupational setting are generally at continued risk for HBV exposure, they should receive the hepatitis B vaccine series.

Safety of PEP for HBV. Hepatitis B vaccines have been found to be safe when administered to infants, children, or adults (*12,50*). Through the year 2000, approximately 100 million persons have received hepatitis B vaccine in the United States. The most common side effects from hepatitis B vaccination are pain at the injection site and mild to moderate fever (*50--55*). Studies indicate that these side effects are reported no more frequently among persons vaccinated than among those receiving placebo (*51,52*).

Approximately 45 reports have been received by the Vaccine Adverse Event Reporting System (VAERS) of alopecia (hair loss) in children and adults after administration of plasma-derived and recombinant hepatitis B vaccine; four persons sustained hair loss following vaccination on more than one occasion (*56*). Hair loss was temporary for approximately two thirds of persons who experienced hair loss. An epidemiologic study conducted in the Vaccine Safety Datalink found no statistical association between alopecia and receipt of hepatitis B vaccine in children (CDC, unpublished data, 1998). A low rate of anaphylaxis has been observed in vaccine recipients based on reports to VAERS; the estimated incidence is 1 in 600,000 vaccine doses distributed. Although none of the persons who developed anaphylaxis died, anaphylactic reactions can be life-threatening; therefore, further vaccination with hepatitis B vaccine is contraindicated in persons with a history of anaphylaxis after a previous dose of vaccine.

Hepatitis B immunization programs conducted on a large scale in Taiwan, Alaska, and New Zealand have observed no association between vaccination and the occurrence of serious adverse events. Furthermore, in the United States, surveillance of adverse events following hepatitis B vaccination has demonstrated no association between hepatitis B vaccine and the occurrence of serious adverse events, including Guillain-Barré syndrome, transverse myelitis, multiple sclerosis, optic neuritis, and seizures (*57--59*) (CDC, unpublished data, 1991). However, several case reports and case series have claimed an association between hepatitis B vaccination and such syndromes and diseases as multiple sclerosis, optic neuritis, rheumatoid arthritis, and other autoimmune diseases (*57,60--66*). Most of these reported adverse events have occurred in adults, and no report has compared the frequency of the purported vaccine-associated syndrome/disease with the frequency in an unvaccinated population. In addition, recent case-control studies have demonstrated no association between hepatitis B vaccination and development or short-term risk of relapse of multiple sclerosis (*67,68*), and reviews by international panels of experts have concluded that available data do not demonstrate a causal association between hepatitis B vaccination and demyelinating diseases, including multiple sclerosis (*69*).

HBIG is prepared from human plasma known to contain a high titer of antibody to HBsAg (anti-HBs). The plasma from which HBIG is prepared is screened for HBsAg and antibodies to HIV and HCV. The process used to prepare HBIG inactivates and eliminates HIV from the final product. Since 1996, the final product has been free of HCV RNA as determined by the polymerase chain reaction (PCR), and, since 1999, all products available in the United States have been manufactured by methods that inactivate HCV and other viruses. No evidence exists that HBV, HCV, or HIV have ever been transmitted by HBIG commercially available in the United States (70,71).

Serious adverse effects from HBIG when administered as recommended have been rare. Local pain and tenderness at the injection site, urticaria and angioedema might occur; anaphylactic reactions, although rare, have been reported following the injection of human immune globulin (IG) preparations (72). Persons with a history of anaphylactic reaction to IG should not receive HBIG.

PEP for HBV During Pregnancy. No apparent risk exists for adverse effects to developing fetuses when hepatitis B vaccine is administered to pregnant women (CDC, unpublished data, 1990). The vaccine contains noninfectious HBsAg particles and should pose no risk to the fetus. HBV infection during pregnancy might result in severe disease for the mother and chronic infection for the newborn. Therefore, neither pregnancy nor lactation should be considered a contraindication to vaccination of women. HBIG is not contraindicated for pregnant or lactating women.

Occupational Transmission of HCV

Risk for Occupational Transmission of HCV

HCV is not transmitted efficiently through occupational exposures to blood. The average incidence of anti-HCV seroconversion after accidental percutaneous exposure from an HCV-positive source is 1.8% (range: 0%--7%) (73--76), with one study indicating that transmission occurred only from hollow-bore needles compared with other sharps (75). Transmission rarely occurs from mucous membrane exposures to blood, and no transmission in HCP has been documented from intact or nonintact skin exposures to blood (77,78). Data are limited on survival of HCV in the environment. In contrast to HBV, the epidemiologic data for HCV suggest that environmental contamination with blood containing HCV is not a significant risk for transmission in the health-care setting (79,80), with the possible exception of the hemodialysis setting where HCV transmission related to environmental contamination and poor infection-control practices have been implicated (81--84). The risk for transmission from exposure to fluids or tissues other than HCV-infected blood also has not been quantified but is expected to be low.

Postexposure Management for HCV

In several studies, researchers have attempted to assess the effectiveness of IG following possible exposure to non-A, non-B hepatitis. These studies have been difficult to interpret because they lack uniformity in diagnostic criteria and study design, and, in all but one study, the first dose of IG was administered before potential exposure (48,85,86). In an experiment designed to model HCV transmission by needlestick exposure in the health-care setting, high anti-HCV titer IG administered to chimpanzees 1 hour after exposure to HCV-positive blood did not prevent transmission of infection (87). In 1994, the Advisory Committee on Immunization Practices (ACIP) reviewed available data regarding the

202

prevention of HCV infection with IG and concluded that using IG as PEP for hepatitis C was not supported (*88*). This conclusion was based on the following facts:

- No protective antibody response has been identified following HCV infection.
- Previous studies of IG use to prevent posttransfusion non-A, non-B hepatitis might not be relevant in making recommendations regarding PEP for hepatitis C.
- Experimental studies in chimpanzees with IG containing anti-HCV failed to prevent transmission of infection after exposure.

No clinical trials have been conducted to assess postexposure use of antiviral agents (e.g., interferon with or without ribavirin) to prevent HCV infection, and antivirals are not FDA-approved for this indication. Available data suggest that an established infection might need to be present before interferon can be an effective treatment. Kinetic studies suggest that the effect of interferon on chronic HCV infection occurs in two phases. During the first phase, interferon blocks the production or release of virus from infected cells. In the second phase, virus is eradicated from the infected cells (*89*); in this later phase, higher pretreatment alanine aminotransferase (ALT) levels correlate with an increasing decline in infected cells, and the rapidity of the decline correlates with viral clearance. In contrast, the effect of antiretrovirals when used for PEP after exposure to HIV is based on inhibition of HIV DNA synthesis early in the retroviral replicative cycle.

In the absence of PEP for HCV, recommendations for postexposure management are intended to achieve early identification of chronic disease and, if present, referral for evaluation of treatment options. However, a theoretical argument is that intervention with antivirals when HCV RNA first becomes detectable might prevent the development of chronic infection. Data from studies conducted outside the United States suggest that a short course of interferon started early in the course of acute hepatitis C is associated with a higher rate of resolved infection than that achieved when therapy is begun after chronic hepatitis C has been well established (*90--92*). These studies used various treatment regimens and included persons with acute disease whose peak ALT levels were 500--1,000 IU/L at the time therapy was initiated (2.6--4 months after exposure).

No studies have evaluated the treatment of acute infection in persons with no evidence of liver disease (i.e., HCV RNA-positive <6 months duration with normal ALT levels); among patients with chronic HCV infection, the efficacy of antivirals has been demonstrated only among patients who also had evidence of chronic liver disease (i.e., abnormal ALT levels). In addition, treatment started early in the course of chronic HCV infection (i.e., 6 months after onset of infection) might be as effective as treatment started during acute infection (*13*). Because 15%--25% of patients with acute HCV infection spontaneously resolve their infection (*93*), treatment of these patients during the acute phase could expose them unnecessarily to the discomfort and side effects of antiviral therapy.

Data upon which to base a recommendation for therapy of acute infection are insufficient because a) no data exist regarding the effect of treating patients with acute infection who have no evidence of disease, b) treatment started early in the course of chronic infection might be just as effective and would eliminate the need to treat persons who will spontaneously resolve their infection, and c) the appropriate regimen is unknown.

Occupational Transmission of HIV

Risk for Occupational Transmission of HIV

In prospective studies of HCP, the average risk of HIV transmission after a percutaneous exposure to HIV-infected blood has been estimated to be approximately 0.3% (95% confidence interval [CI] = 0.2%--0.5%) (94) and after a mucous membrane exposure, approximately 0.09% (95% CI = 0.006%--0.5%) (95). Although episodes of HIV transmission after nonintact skin exposure have been documented (96), the average risk for transmission by this route has not been precisely quantified but is estimated to be less than the risk for mucous membrane exposures (97). The risk for transmission after exposure to fluids or tissues other than HIV-infected blood also has not been quantified but is probably considerably lower than for blood exposures (98).

As of June 2000, CDC had received voluntary reports of 56 U.S. HCP with documented HIV seroconversion temporally associated with an occupational HIV exposure. An additional 138 episodes in HCP are considered possible occupational HIV transmissions. These workers had a history of occupational exposure to blood, other infectious body fluids, or laboratory solutions containing HIV, and no other risk for HIV infection was identified, but HIV seroconversion after a specific exposure was not documented (99).

Epidemiologic and laboratory studies suggest that several factors might affect the risk of HIV transmission after an occupational exposure. In a retrospective case-control study of HCP who had percutaneous exposure to HIV, the risk for HIV infection was found to be increased with exposure to a larger quantity of blood from the source person as indicated by a) a device visibly contaminated with the patient's blood, b) a procedure that involved a needle being placed directly in a vein or artery, or c) a deep injury (100). The risk also was increased for exposure to blood from source persons with terminal illness, possibly reflecting either the higher titer of HIV in blood late in the course of AIDS or other factors (e.g., the presence of syncytia-inducing strains of HIV). A laboratory study that demonstrated that more blood is transferred by deeper injuries and hollow-bore needles lends further support for the observed variation in risk related to blood quantity (101).

The use of source person viral load as a surrogate measure of viral titer for assessing transmission risk has not yet been established. Plasma viral load (e.g., HIV RNA) reflects only the level of cell-free virus in the peripheral blood; latently infected cells might transmit infection in the absence of viremia. Although a lower viral load (e.g., <1,500 RNA copies/mL) or one that is below the limits of detection probably indicates a lower titer exposure, it does not rule out the possibility of transmission.

Some evidence exists regarding host defenses possibly influencing the risk for HIV infection. A study of HIV-exposed but uninfected HCP demonstrated an HIV-specific cytotoxic T-lymphocyte (CTL) response when peripheral blood mononuclear cells were stimulated in vitro with HIV-specific antigens (*102*). Similar CTL responses have been observed in other groups who experienced repeated HIV exposure without resulting infection (*103--108*). Among several possible explanations for this observation is that the host immune response sometimes might prevent establishment of HIV infection after a percutaneous exposure; another is that the CTL response simply might be a marker for exposure. In a study of 20 HCP with occupational exposure to HIV, a comparison was made of HCP treated with zidovudine (ZDV) PEP and those not treated. The findings from this study suggest that ZDV blunted the HIV-specific CTL response and that PEP might inhibit early HIV replication (*109*).

Rationale for HIV PEP

Considerations that influence the rationale and recommendations for PEP include

- the pathogenesis of HIV infection, particularly the time course of early infection;
- the biological plausibility that infection can be prevented or ameliorated by using antiretroviral drugs;
- direct or indirect evidence of the efficacy of specific agents used for prophylaxis; and
- the risk and benefit of PEP to exposed HCP.

The following discussion considers each of these concerns.

Role of Pathogenesis in Considering Antiretroviral Prophylaxis. Information about primary HIV infection indicates that systemic infection does not occur immediately, leaving a brief window of opportunity during which postexposure antiretroviral intervention might modify or prevent viral replication. In a primate model of simian immunodeficiency virus (SIV) infection, infection of dendritic-like cells occurred at the site of inoculation during the first 24 hours following mucosal exposure to cell-free virus. Over the subsequent 24--48 hours, migration of these cells to regional lymph nodes occurred, and virus was detectable in the peripheral blood within 5 days (*110*). Theoretically, initiation of antiretroviral PEP soon after exposure might prevent or inhibit systemic infection by limiting the proliferation of virus in the initial target cells or lymph nodes.

Efficacy of Antiretrovirals for PEP in Animal Studies. Data from animal studies have been difficult to interpret, in part, because of problems identifying an animal model that is comparable to humans. In early studies, differences in controlled variables (e.g., choice of viral strain [based on the animal model used], inoculum size, route of inoculation, time of prophylaxis initiation, and drug regimen) made extrapolation of the results to humans difficult. Recently, refinements in methodology have facilitated more relevant studies; in particular, the viral inocula used in animal studies have been reduced to levels more analogous to human exposures but sufficient to cause infection in control animals (*111--113*). These studies provide encouraging evidence of postexposure chemoprophylactic efficacy.

Studies among primates and in murine and feline animal models have demonstrated that larger viral inocula decrease prophylactic efficacy (*114--117*). In addition, delaying initiation, shortening the duration, or decreasing the antiretroviral dose of PEP, individually or in combination, decreased prophylactic efficacy (*113,118--124*). For example, when (R)-9-(2-phosphonylmethoxypropyl) adenine (tenofovir) was administered 48 hours before, 4 hours after, or 24 hours after intravenous SIV inoculation to long-tailed macaques, a 4-week regimen prevented infection in all treated animals (*122*). A subsequent study confirmed the efficacy of tenofovir PEP when administered 24 hours after intravenous inoculation of a dose of SIV that uniformly results in infection in untreated macaques. In the same study, protection was incomplete if the tenofovir administration was delayed to 48 or 72 hours postexposure or if the total duration of treatment was curtailed to 3 or 10 days (*123*).

Efficacy of Antiretrovirals for PEP in Human Studies. Little information exists from which the efficacy of PEP in humans can be assessed. Seroconversion is infrequent following an occupational exposure to HIV-infected blood; therefore, several thousands of exposed HCP would need to enroll in a prospective trial to achieve the statistical power necessary to directly demonstrate PEP efficacy (*125*).

In the retrospective case-control study of HCP, after controlling for other risk factors for HIV transmission, use of ZDV as PEP was associated with a reduction in the risk of HIV infection by approximately 81% (95% CI = 43%--94%) (*100*). Although the results of this study suggest PEP efficacy, its limitations include the small number of cases studied and the use of cases and controls from different cohorts.

In a multicenter trial in which ZDV was administered to HIV-infected pregnant women and their infants, the administration of ZDV during pregnancy, labor, and delivery and to the infant reduced transmission by 67% (*126*). Only part of the protective effect of ZDV was explained by reduction of the HIV viral load in the maternal blood, suggesting that ZDV prophylaxis, in part, involves a mechanism other than the reduction of maternal viral burden (*127,128*). Since 1998, studies have highlighted the importance of PEP for prevention of perinatal HIV transmission. In Africa, the use of ZDV in combination with lamivudine (3TC) decreased perinatal HIV transmission by 50% when administered during pregnancy, labor, and for 1 week postpartum, and by 37% when started at the onset of labor and continued for 1 week postpartum (*129*). Studies in the United States and Uganda also have demonstrated that rates of perinatal HIV transmission have been reduced with the use of abbreviated PEP regimens started intrapartum or during the first 48--72 hours of life (*130--132*).

The limitations of all of these studies with animals and humans must be considered when reviewing evidence of PEP efficacy. The extent to which data from animal studies can be extrapolated to humans is largely unknown, and the exposure route for mother-to-infant HIV transmission is not similar to occupational exposures; therefore, these findings might not be directly applicable to PEP in HCP.

Reports of Failure of PEP. Failure of PEP to prevent HIV infection in HCP has been reported in at least 21 instances (*78,133--139*). In 16 of the cases, ZDV was used alone as a single agent; in two cases, ZDV and didanosine (ddI) were used in combination (*133,138*); and in three cases, ≥3 drugs were used for PEP (*137--139*). Thirteen of the source persons were known to have been treated with antiretroviral therapy before the exposure. Antiretroviral resistance testing of the virus from the source person was performed in seven instances, and in four, the HIV infection transmitted was found to have decreased sensitivity to ZDV and/or other drugs used for PEP. In addition to possible exposure to an antiretroviral-resistant strain of HIV, other factors that might have contributed to these apparent failures might include a high titer and/or large inoculum exposure, delayed initiation and/or short duration of PEP, and possible factors related to the host (e.g., cellular immune system responsiveness) and/or to the source person's virus (e.g., presence of syncytia-forming strains) (*133*). Details regarding the cases of PEP failure involving combinations of antiretroviral agents are included in this report (Table 1).

Antiretroviral Agents for PEP

Antiretroviral agents from three classes of drugs are available for the treatment of HIV infection. These agents include the nucleoside reverse transcriptase inhibitors (NRTIs), nonnucleoside reverse transcriptase inhibitors (NNRTIs), and protease inhibitors (PIs). Only antiretroviral agents that have been approved by FDA for treatment of HIV infection are discussed in these guidelines.

Determining which agents and how many to use or when to alter a PEP regimen is largely empiric. Guidelines for the treatment of HIV infection, a condition usually involving a high total body burden of HIV, include recommendations for the use of three drugs (*140*); however, the applicability of these recommendations to PEP remains unknown. In HIV-infected patients, combination regimens have proved superior to monotherapy regimens in reducing HIV viral load, reducing the incidence of opportunistic infections and death, and delaying onset of drug resistance (*141,142*). A combination of drugs with activity at different stages in the viral replication cycle (e.g., nucleoside analogues with a PI) theoretically could offer an additional preventive effect in PEP, particularly for occupational exposures that pose an increased risk of transmission. Although the use of a three-drug regimen might be justified for exposures that pose an increased risk of transmission, whether the potential added toxicity of a third drug is justified for lower-risk exposures is uncertain. Therefore, the recommendations at the end of this document provide guidance for two- and three-drug PEP regimens that are based on the level of risk for HIV transmission represented by the exposure.

NRTI combinations that can be considered for PEP include ZDV and 3TC, 3TC and stavudine (d4T), and ddI and d4T. In previous PHS guidelines, a combination of ZDV and 3TC was considered the first choice for PEP regimens (*3*). Because ZDV and 3TC are available in a combination formulation (Combivir™, manufactured by Glaxo Wellcome, Inc., Research Triangle Park, NC), the use of this combination might be more convenient for HCP. However, recent data suggest that mutations associated with ZDV and 3TC resistance might be common in some areas (*143*). Thus, individual clinicians might prefer other NRTIs or combinations based on local knowledge and experience in treating HIV infection and disease.

The addition of a third drug for PEP following high-risk exposures is based on demonstrated effectiveness in reducing viral burden in HIV-infected persons. Previously, indinavir (IDV) or nelfinavir (NFV) were recommended as first-choice agents for inclusion in an expanded PEP regimen (*5*). Since the publication of the 1998 PEP guidelines, efavirenz (EFV), an NNRTI; abacavir (ABC), a potent NRTI; and Kaletra™, a PI, have been approved by FDA. Although side effects might be common with the NNRTIs, EFV might be considered for expanded PEP regimens, especially when resistance to PIs in the source person's virus is known or suspected. ABC has been associated with dangerous hypersensitivity reactions but, with careful monitoring, may be considered as a third drug for PEP. Kaletra, a combination of lopinavir and ritonavir, is a potent HIV inhibitor that, with expert consultation, may be considered in an expanded PEP regimen.

Toxicity and Drug Interactions of Antiretroviral Agents. When administering PEP, an important goal is completion of a 4-week PEP regimen when PEP is indicated. Therefore, the toxicity profile of antiretroviral agents, including the frequency, severity, duration, and reversibility of side effects, is a relevant consideration. All of the antiretroviral agents have been associated with side effects (Table 2). However, studies of adverse events have been conducted primarily with persons who have advanced disease (and longer treatment courses) and who therefore might not reflect the experience in persons who are uninfected (*144*).

Several primary side effects are associated with antiretroviral agents (Table 2). Side effects associated with many of the NRTIs are chiefly gastrointestinal (e.g., nausea or diarrhea); however, ddI has been associated with cases of fatal and nonfatal pancreatitis among HIV-infected patients treated for >4 weeks. The use of PIs has been associated with new onset diabetes mellitus, hyperglycemia, diabetic ketoacidosis, exacerbation of preexisting diabetes mellitus, and dyslipidemia (*145--147*). Nephrolithiasis has been associated with IDV use; however, the incidence of this potential complication might be limited by drinking at least 48 ounces (1.5 L) of fluid per 24-hour period (e.g., six 8-ounce glasses of water throughout the day) (*148*). NFV has been associated with the development of diarrhea; however, this side effect might respond to treatment with antimotility agents that can be prescribed for use, if necessary, at the time the drug is recommended for PEP. The NNRTIs have been associated with severe skin reactions, including life-threatening cases of Stevens-Johnson syndrome and toxic epidermal necrolysis. Hepatotoxicity, including fatal hepatic necrosis, has occurred in patients treated with nevirapine (NVP); some episodes began during the first few weeks of therapy (FDA, unpublished data, 2000). EFV has been associated with central nervous system side effects, including dizziness, somnolence, insomnia, and abnormal dreaming.

All of the approved antiretroviral agents might have potentially serious drug interactions when used with certain other drugs (Appendix C). Careful evaluation of concomitant medications used by an exposed person is required before PEP is prescribed, and close monitoring for toxicity is also needed. Further information about potential drug interactions can be found in the manufacturer's package insert.

Toxicity Associated with PEP. Information from the National Surveillance System for Health Care Workers (NaSH) and the HIV Postexposure Registry indicates that nearly 50% of HCP experience adverse symptoms (e.g., nausea, malaise, headache, anorexia, and headache) while taking PEP and that approximately 33% stop taking PEP because of adverse signs and symptoms (*6,7,10,11*). Some studies have demonstrated that side effects and discontinuation of PEP are more common among HCP taking three-drug combination regimens for PEP compared with HCP taking two-drug combination regimens (*7,10*). Although similar rates of side effects were observed among persons who took PEP after sexual or drug use exposures to HIV in the San Francisco Post-Exposure Prevention Project, 80% completed 4 weeks of therapy (*149*). Participants in the San Francisco Project were followed at 1, 2, 4, 26, and 52 weeks postexposure and received medication adherence counseling; most participants took only two drugs for PEP.

Serious side effects, including nephrolithiasis, hepatitis, and pancytopenia have been reported with the use of combination drugs for PEP (*6,7,150,151*). One case of NVP-associated fulminant liver failure requiring liver transplantation and one case of hypersensitivity syndrome have been reported in HCP taking NVP for HIV PEP (*152*). Including these two cases, from March 1997 through September 2000, FDA received reports of 22 cases of serious adverse events related to NVP taken for PEP (*153*). These events included 12 cases of hepatotoxicity, 14 cases of skin reaction (including one documented and two possible cases of Stevens-Johnson syndrome), and one case of rhabdomyolysis; four cases involved both hepatotoxicty and skin reaction, and one case involved both rhabdomyolysis and skin reaction.

Resistance to Antiretroviral Agents. Known or suspected resistance of the source virus to antiretroviral agents, particularly to agents that might be included in a PEP regimen, is a concern for persons making decisions about PEP. Resistance to HIV infection occurs with all of the available antiretroviral agents, and cross-resistance within drug classes is frequent (*154*). Recent studies have demonstrated an emergence of drug-resistant HIV among source persons for occupational exposures (*143,155*). A study conducted at seven U.S. sites during 1998--1999 found that 16 (39%) of 41 source persons whose virus was sequenced had primary genetic mutations associated with resistance to RTIs, and 4 (10%) had primary mutations associated with resistance to PIs (*143*). In addition, occupational transmission of resistant HIV strains, despite PEP with combination drug regimens, has been reported (*137,139*). In one case, a hospital worker became infected after an HIV exposure despite a PEP regimen that included ddI, d4T, and NVP (*139*). The transmitted HIV contained two primary genetic mutations associated with resistance to NNRTIs (the source person was taking EFV at the time of the exposure). Despite recent studies and case reports, the relevance of exposure to a resistant virus is still not well understood.

Empiric decisions about the presence of antiretroviral drug resistance are often difficult to make because patients generally take more than one antiretroviral agent. Resistance should be suspected in source persons when they are experiencing clinical progression of disease or a persistently increasing viral load, and/or decline in CD4 T-cell count, despite therapy or a lack of virologic response to therapy. However, resistance testing of the source virus at the time of an exposure is not practical because the results will not be available in time to influence the choice of the initial PEP regimen. Furthermore, in this situation, whether modification of the PEP regimen is necessary or will influence the outcome of an occupational exposure is unknown. No data exist to suggest that modification of a PEP regimen after receiving results from resistance testing (usually a minimum of 1--2 weeks) improves efficacy of PEP.

Antiretroviral Drugs During Pregnancy. Data are limited on the potential effects of antiretroviral drugs on the developing fetus or neonate (*156*). Carcinogenicity and/or mutagenicity is evident in several in vitro screening tests for ZDV and all other FDA-licensed NRTIs. The relevance of animal data to humans is unknown; however, because teratogenic effects were observed in primates at drug exposures similar to those representing human therapeutic exposure, the use of EFV should be avoided in pregnant women (*140*). IDV is associated with infrequent side effects in adults (i.e., hyperbilirubinemia and renal stones) that could be problematic for a newborn. Because the half-life of IDV in adults is short, these concerns might be relevant only if the drug is administered shortly before delivery.

In a recent study in France of perinatal HIV transmission, two cases of progressive neurologic disease and death were reported in uninfected infants exposed to ZDV and 3TC (*157*). Laboratory studies of these children suggested mitochondrial dysfunction. In a careful review of deaths in children followed in U.S. perinatal HIV cohorts, no deaths attributable to mitochondrial disease have been found (*158*).

Recent reports of fatal and nonfatal lactic acidosis in pregnant women treated throughout gestation with a combination of d4T and ddI have prompted warnings about use of these drugs during pregnancy (*159*). Although the case-patients were HIV-infected women taking the drugs for >4 weeks, pregnant women and their providers should be advised to consider d4T and ddI only when the benefits of their use outweigh the risks.

PEP Use in Hospitals in the United States. Analysis of data from NaSH provides information on the use of PEP following occupational exposures in 47 hospitals in the United States. A total of 11,784 exposures to blood and body fluids was reported from June 1996 through November 2000 (CDC, unpublished data, 2001). For all exposures with known sources, 6% were to HIV-positive sources, 74% to HIV-negative sources, and 20% to sources with an unknown HIV status. Sixty-three percent of HCP exposed to a known HIV-positive source started PEP, and 54% of HCP took it for at least 20 days, whereas 14% of HCP exposed to a source person subsequently found to be HIV-negative initiated PEP, and 3% of those took it for at least 20 days. Information recorded about HIV exposures in NaSH indicates that 46% of exposures involving an HIV-positive source warranted only a two-drug PEP regimen (i.e., the exposure was to mucous membranes or skin or was a superficial percutaneous injury and the source person did not have end-stage AIDS or acute HIV illness); however, 53% of these exposed HCP took ≥3 drugs (CDC, unpublished data, 2000). Similarly, the National Clinicians' Post-Exposure Prophylaxis Hotline (PEPline) reported that PEPline staff recommended stopping or not starting PEP for approximately one half of the HCP who consulted them about exposures (D. Bangsberg, San Francisco General Hospital, unpublished data, September 1999). The observation that some HCP exposed to HIV-negative source persons take PEP from several days to weeks following their exposures suggests that strategies be employed such as the use of a rapid HIV antibody assay, which could minimize exposure to unnecessary PEP (11). A recent study demonstrated that use of a rapid HIV test for evaluation of source persons after occupational exposures not only resulted in decreased use of PEP, but also was cost-effective compared with use of the standard enzyme immunoassay (EIA) test for source persons subsequently found to be HIV-negative (160).

RECOMMENDATIONS FOR THE MANAGEMENT OF HCP POTENTIALLY EXPOSED TO HBV, HCV, or HIV

Exposure prevention remains the primary strategy for reducing occupational bloodborne pathogen infections; however, occupational exposures will continue to occur. Health-care organizations should make available to their personnel a system that includes written protocols for prompt reporting, evaluation, counseling, treatment, and follow-up of occupational exposures that might place HCP at risk for acquiring a bloodborne infection. HCP should be educated concerning the risk for and prevention of bloodborne infections, including the need to be vaccinated against hepatitis B (17,21,161--163). Employers are required to establish exposure-control plans that include postexposure follow-up for their employees and to comply with incident reporting requirements mandated by the 1992 OSHA bloodborne pathogen standard (2). Access to clinicians who can provide postexposure care should be available during all working hours, including nights and weekends. HBIG, hepatitis B vaccine, and antiretroviral agents for HIV PEP should be available for timely administration (i.e., either by providing access on-site or by creating linkages with other facilities or providers to make them available off-site). Persons responsible for providing postexposure management should be familiar with evaluation and treatment protocols and the facility's plans for accessing HBIG, hepatitis B vaccine, and antiretroviral drugs for HIV PEP.

HCP should be educated to report occupational exposures immediately after they occur, particularly because HBIG, hepatitis B vaccine, and HIV PEP are most likely to be effective if administered as soon after the exposure as possible. HCP who are at risk for occupational exposure to bloodborne pathogens should be familiarized with the principles of postexposure management as part of job orientation and ongoing job training.

Hepatitis B Vaccination

Any person who performs tasks involving contact with blood, blood-contaminated body fluids, other body fluids, or sharps should be vaccinated against hepatitis B (2,21). Prevaccination serologic screening for previous infection is not indicated for persons being vaccinated because of occupational risk, unless the hospital or health-care organization considers screening cost-effective.

Hepatitis B vaccine should always be administered by the intramuscular route in the deltoid muscle with a needle 1--1.5 inches long. Hepatitis B vaccine can be administered at the same time as other vaccines with no interference with antibody response to the other vaccines (164). If the vaccination series is interrupted after the first dose, the second dose should be administered as soon as possible. The second and third doses should be separated by an interval of at least 2 months. If only the third dose is delayed, it should be administered when convenient. HCP who have contact with patients or blood and are at ongoing risk for percutaneous injuries should be tested 1--2 months after completion of the 3dose vaccination series for anti-HBs (21). Persons who do not respond to the primary vaccine series (i.e., anti-HBs <10 mIU/mL) should complete a second 3-dose vaccine series or be evaluated to determine if they are HBsAg-positive. Revaccinated persons should be retested at the completion of the second vaccine series. Persons who do not respond to an initial 3-dose vaccine series have a 30%--50% chance of responding to a second 3-dose series (165). Persons who prove to be HBsAg-positive should be counseled regarding how to prevent HBV transmission to others and regarding the need for medical evaluation (12,163,166). Nonresponders to vaccination who are HBsAg-negative should be considered susceptible to HBV infection and should be counseled regarding precautions to prevent HBV infection and the need to obtain HBIG prophylaxis for any known or probable parenteral exposure to HBsAg-positive blood. Booster doses of hepatitis B vaccine are not necessary, and periodic serologic testing to monitor antibody concentrations after completion of the vaccine series is not recommended. Any blood or body fluid exposure sustained by an unvaccinated, susceptible person should lead to the initiation of the hepatitis B vaccine series.

Treatment of an Exposure Site

Wounds and skin sites that have been in contact with blood or body fluids should be washed with soap and water; mucous membranes should be flushed with water. No evidence exists that using antiseptics for wound care or expressing fluid by squeezing the wound further reduces the risk of bloodborne pathogen transmission; however, the use of antiseptics is not contraindicated. The application of caustic agents (e.g., bleach) or the injection of antiseptics or disinfectants into the wound is not recommended.

Exposure Report

If an occupational exposure occurs, the circumstances and postexposure management should be recorded in the exposed person's confidential medical record (usually on a form the facility designates for this purpose) (Box 1). In addition, employers should follow all federal (including OSHA) and state requirements for recording and reporting occupational injuries and exposures.

Evaluation of the Exposure and the Exposure Source

Evaluation of the Exposure

The exposure should be evaluated for the potential to transmit HBV, HCV, and HIV based on the type of body substance involved and the route and severity of the exposure (Box 2). Blood, fluid containing visible blood, or other potentially infectious fluid (including semen; vaginal secretions; and cerebrospinal, synovial, pleural, peritoneal, pericardial, and amniotic fluids) or tissue can be infectious for bloodborne viruses. Exposures to these fluids or tissue through a percutaneous injury (i.e., needlestick or other penetrating sharps-related event) or through contact with a mucous membrane are situations that pose a risk for bloodborne virus transmission and require further evaluation. For HCV and HIV, exposure to a blood-filled hollow needle or visibly bloody device suggests a higher risk exposure than exposure to a needle that was most likely used for giving an injection. In addition, any direct contact (i.e, personal protective equipment either was not present or was ineffective in protecting skin or mucous membranes) with concentrated virus in a research laboratory or production facility is considered an exposure that requires clinical evaluation.

For skin exposure, follow-up is indicated only if it involves exposure to a body fluid previously listed and evidence exists of compromised skin integrity (e.g., dermatitis, abrasion, or open wound). In the clinical evaluation for human bites, possible exposure of both the person bitten and the person who inflicted the bite must be considered. If a bite results in blood exposure to either person involved, postexposure follow-up should be provided.

Evaluation of the Exposure Source

The person whose blood or body fluid is the source of an occupational exposure should be evaluated for HBV, HCV, and HIV infection (Box 3). Information available in the medical record at the time of exposure (e.g., laboratory test results, admitting diagnosis, or previous medical history) or from the source person, might confirm or exclude bloodborne virus infection.

If the HBV, HCV, and/or HIV infection status of the source is unknown, the source person should be informed of the incident and tested for serologic evidence of bloodborne virus infection. Procedures should be followed for testing source persons, including obtaining informed consent, in accordance with applicable state and local laws. Any persons determined to be infected with HBV, HCV, or HIV should be referred for appropriate counseling and treatment. Confidentiality of the source person should be maintained at all times.

Testing to determine the HBV, HCV, and HIV infection status of an exposure source should be performed as soon as possible. Hospitals, clinics and other sites that manage exposed HCP should consult their laboratories regarding the most appropriate test to use to expedite obtaining these results. An FDA-approved rapid HIV-antibody test kit should be considered for use in this situation, particularly if testing by EIA cannot be completed within 24--48 hours. Repeatedly reactive results by EIA or rapid HIV-antibody tests are considered to be highly suggestive of infection, whereas a negative result is an excellent indicator of the absence of HIV antibody. Confirmation of a reactive result by Western blot or immunofluorescent antibody is not necessary to make initial decisions about postexposure management but should be done to complete the testing process and before informing the source person. Repeatedly reactive results by EIA for anti-HCV should be confirmed by a supplemental test (i.e., recombinant immunoblot assay [RIBA™] or HCV PCR). Direct virus assays (e.g., HIV p24 antigen EIA or tests for HIV RNA or HCV RNA) for routine HIV or HCV screening of source persons are not recommended.

If the exposure source is unknown or cannot be tested, information about where and under what circumstances the exposure occurred should be assessed epidemiologically for the likelihood of transmission of HBV, HCV, or HIV. Certain situations as well as the type of exposure might suggest an increased or decreased risk; an important consideration is the prevalence of HBV, HCV, or HIV in the population group (i.e., institution or community) from which the contaminated source material is derived. For example, an exposure that occurs in a geographic area where injection-drug use is prevalent or involves a needle discarded in a drug-treatment facility would be considered epidemiologically to have a higher risk for transmission than an exposure that occurs in a nursing home for the elderly.

Testing of needles or other sharp instruments implicated in an exposure, regardless of whether the source is known or unknown, is not recommended. The reliability and interpretation of findings in such circumstances are unknown, and testing might be hazardous to persons handling the sharp instrument.

Examples of information to consider when evaluating an exposure source for possible HBV, HCV, or HIV infection include laboratory information (e.g., previous HBV, HCV, or HIV test results or results of immunologic testing [e.g., CD4+ T-cell count]) or liver enzymes (e.g., ALT), clinical symptoms (e.g., acute syndrome suggestive of primary HIV infection or undiagnosed immunodeficiency disease), and history of recent (i.e., within 3 months) possible HBV, HCV, or HIV exposures (e.g., injection-drug use or sexual contact with a known positive partner). Health-care providers should be aware of local and state laws governing the collection and release of HIV serostatus information on a source person, following an occupational exposure.

If the source person is known to have HIV infection, available information about this person's stage of infection (i.e., asymptomatic, symptomatic, or AIDS), CD4+ T-cell count, results of viral load testing, current and previous antiretroviral therapy, and results of any genotypic or phenotypic viral resistance testing should be gathered for consideration in choosing an appropriate PEP regimen. If this information is not immediately available, initiation of PEP, if indicated, should not be delayed; changes in the PEP regimen can be made after PEP has been started, as appropriate. Reevaluation of exposed HCP should be considered within 72 hours postexposure, especially as additional information about the exposure or source person becomes available.

If the source person is HIV seronegative and has no clinical evidence of AIDS or symptoms of HIV infection, no further testing of the person for HIV infection is indicated. The likelihood of the source person being in the "window period" of HIV infection in the absence of symptoms of acute retroviral syndrome is extremely small.

Management of Exposures to HBV

For percutaneous or mucosal exposures to blood, several factors must be considered when making a decision to provide prophylaxis, including the HBsAg status of the source and the hepatitis B vaccination and vaccine-response status of the exposed person. Such exposures usually involve persons for whom hepatitis B vaccination is recommended. Any blood or body fluid exposure to an unvaccinated person should lead to initiation of the hepatitis B vaccine series.

The hepatitis B vaccination status and the vaccine-response status (if known) of the exposed person should be reviewed. A summary of prophylaxis recommendations for percutaneous or mucosal exposure to blood according to the HBsAg status of the exposure source and the vaccination and vaccine-response status of the exposed person is included in this report (Table 3).

When HBIG is indicated, it should be administered as soon as possible after exposure (preferably within 24 hours). The effectiveness of HBIG when administered >7 days after exposure is unknown. When hepatitis B vaccine is indicated, it should also be administered as soon as possible (preferably within 24 hours) and can be administered simultaneously with HBIG at a separate site (vaccine should always be administered in the deltoid muscle).

For exposed persons who are in the process of being vaccinated but have not completed the vaccination series, vaccination should be completed as scheduled, and HBIG should be added as indicated (Table 3). Persons exposed to HBsAg-positive blood or body fluids who are known not to have responded to a primary vaccine series should receive a single dose of HBIG and reinitiate the hepatitis B vaccine series with the first dose of the hepatitis B vaccine as soon as possible after exposure. Alternatively, they should receive two doses of HBIG, one dose as soon as possible after exposure, and the second dose 1 month later. The option of administering one dose of HBIG and reinitiating the vaccine series is preferred for nonresponders who did not complete a second 3-dose vaccine series. For persons who previously completed a second vaccine series but failed to respond, two doses of HBIG are preferred.

Management of Exposures to HCV

Individual institutions should establish policies and procedures for testing HCP for HCV after percutaneous or mucosal exposures to blood and ensure that all personnel are familiar with these policies and procedures. The following are recommendations for follow-up of occupational HCV exposures:

215

- For the source, perform testing for anti-HCV.
- For the person exposed to an HCV-positive source

    --- perform baseline testing for anti-HCV and ALT activity; and

    --- perform follow-up testing (e.g., at 4--6 months) for anti-HCV and ALT activity (if earlier diagnosis of HCV infection is desired, testing for HCV RNA may be performed at 4--6 weeks).

- Confirm all anti-HCV results reported positive by enzyme immunoassay using supplemental anti-HCV testing (e.g., recombinant immunoblot assay [RIBA™]) (13).

Health-care professionals who provide care to persons exposed to HCV in the occupational setting should be knowledgeable regarding the risk for HCV infection and appropriate counseling, testing, and medical follow-up.

IG and antiviral agents are not recommended for PEP after exposure to HCV-positive blood. In addition, no guidelines exist for administration of therapy during the acute phase of HCV infection. However, limited data indicate that antiviral therapy might be beneficial when started early in the course of HCV infection. When HCV infection is identified early, the person should be referred for medical management to a specialist knowledgeable in this area.

Counseling for HCP Exposed to Viral Hepatitis

HCP exposed to HBV- or HCV-infected blood do not need to take any special precautions to prevent secondary transmission during the follow-up period (12,13); however, they should refrain from donating blood, plasma, organs, tissue, or semen. The exposed person does not need to modify sexual practices or refrain from becoming pregnant. If an exposed woman is breast feeding, she does not need to discontinue.

No modifications to an exposed person's patient-care responsibilities are necessary to prevent transmission to patients based solely on exposure to HBV- or HCV-positive blood. If an exposed person becomes acutely infected with HBV, the person should be evaluated according to published recommendations for infected HCP (165). No recommendations exist regarding restricting the professional activities of HCP with HCV infection (13). As recommended for all HCP, those who are chronically infected with HBV or HCV should follow all recommended infection-control practices, including standard precautions and appropriate use of hand washing, protective barriers, and care in the use and disposal of needles and other sharp instruments (162).

Management of Exposures to HIV

Clinical Evaluation and Baseline Testing of Exposed HCP

HCP exposed to HIV should be evaluated within hours (rather than days) after their exposure and should be tested for HIV at baseline (i.e., to establish infection status at the time of exposure). If the source person is seronegative for HIV, baseline testing or further follow-up of the exposed person normally is not necessary. Serologic testing should be made available to all HCP who are concerned that they might have been occupationally infected with HIV. For purposes of considering HIV PEP, the evaluation also should include information about medications the exposed person might be taking and any current or underlying medical conditions or circumstances (i.e., pregnancy, breast feeding, or renal or hepatic disease) that might influence drug selection.

PEP for HIV

The following recommendations (Table 4 and Table 5) apply to situations when a person has been exposed to a source person with HIV infection or when information suggests the likelihood that the source person is HIV-infected. These recommendations are based on the risk for HIV infection after different types of exposure and on limited data regarding efficacy and toxicity of PEP. Because most occupational HIV exposures do not result in the transmission of HIV, potential toxicity must be carefully considered when prescribing PEP. To assist with the initial management of an HIV exposure, health-care facilities should have drugs for an initial PEP regimen selected and available for use. When possible, these recommendations should be implemented in consultation with persons who have expertise in antiretroviral therapy and HIV transmission (Box 4).

Timing and Duration of PEP. PEP should be initiated as soon as possible. The interval within which PEP should be initiated for optimal efficacy is not known. Animal studies have demonstrated the importance of starting PEP soon after an exposure (*111,112,118*). If questions exist about which antiretroviral drugs to use or whether to use a basic or expanded regimen, starting the basic regimen immediately rather than delaying PEP administration is probably better. Although animal studies suggest that PEP probably is substantially less effective when started more than 24--36 hours postexposure (*112,119,122*), the interval after which no benefit is gained from PEP for humans is undefined. Therefore, if appropriate for the exposure, PEP should be started even when the interval since exposure exceeds 36 hours. Initiating therapy after a longer interval (e.g., 1 week) might be considered for exposures that represent an increased risk for transmission. The optimal duration of PEP is unknown. Because 4 weeks of ZDV appeared protective in occupational and animal studies (*100,123*), PEP probably should be administered for 4 weeks, if tolerated.

Use of PEP When HIV Infection Status of Source Person is Unknown. If the source person's HIV infection status is unknown at the time of exposure, use of PEP should be decided on a case-by-case basis, after considering the type of exposure and the clinical and/or epidemiologic likelihood of HIV infection in the source (Table 4 and Table 5). If these considerations suggest a possibility for HIV transmission and HIV testing of the source person is pending, initiating a two-drug PEP regimen until laboratory results have been obtained and later modifying or discontinuing the regimen accordingly is reasonable. The following are recommendations regarding HIV postexposure prophylaxis:

- If indicated, start PEP as soon as possible after an exposure.
- Reevaluation of the exposed person should be considered within 72 hours postexposure, especially as additional information about the exposure or source person becomes available.
- Administer PEP for 4 weeks, if tolerated.
- If a source person is determined to be HIV-negative, PEP should be discontinued.

PEP for Pregnant HCP. If the exposed person is pregnant, the evaluation of risk of infection and need for PEP should be approached as with any other person who has had an HIV exposure. However, the decision to use any antiretroviral drug during pregnancy should involve discussion between the woman and her health-care provider(s) regarding the potential benefits and risks to her and her fetus.

Certain drugs should be avoided in pregnant women. Because teratogenic effects were observed in primate studies, EFV is not recommended during pregnancy. Reports of fatal lactic acidosis in pregnant women treated with a combination of d4T and ddI have prompted warnings about these drugs during pregnancy. Because of the risk of hyperbilirubinemia in newborns, IDV should not be administered to pregnant women shortly before delivery.

Recommendations for the Selection of Drugs for HIV PEP

Health-care providers must strive to balance the risk for infection against the potential toxicity of the agent(s) used when selecting a drug regimen for HIV PEP. Because PEP is potentially toxic, its use is not justified for exposures that pose a negligible risk for transmission (Table 4 and Table 5). Also, insufficient evidence exists to support recommending a three-drug regimen for all HIV exposures. Therefore, two regimens for PEP are provided (Appendix C): a "basic" two-drug regimen that should be appropriate for most HIV exposures and an "expanded" three-drug regimen that should be used for exposures that pose an increased risk for transmission (Table 4 and Table 5). When possible, the regimens should be implemented in consultation with persons who have expertise in antiretroviral treatment and HIV transmission.

Most HIV exposures will warrant a two-drug regimen using two nucleoside analogues (e.g., ZDV and 3TC; or 3TC and d4T; or d4T and ddI). The addition of a third drug should be considered for exposures that pose an increased risk for transmission. Selection of the PEP regimen should consider the comparative risk represented by the exposure and information about the exposure source, including history of and response to antiretroviral therapy based on clinical response, CD4+ T-cell counts, viral load measurements, and current disease stage. When the source person's virus is known or suspected to be resistant to one or more of the drugs considered for the PEP regimen, the selection of drugs to which the source person's virus is unlikely to be resistant is recommended; expert consultation is advised. If this information is not immediately available, initiation of PEP, if indicated, should not be delayed; changes in the PEP regimen can be made after PEP has been started, as appropriate. Reevaluation of the exposed person should be considered within 72 hours postexposure, especially as additional information about the exposure or source person becomes available.

Follow-up of HCP Exposed to HIV

Postexposure Testing. HCP with occupational exposure to HIV should receive follow-up counseling, postexposure testing, and medical evaluation, regardless of whether they receive PEP. HIV-antibody testing should be performed for at least 6 months postexposure (e.g., at 6 weeks, 12 weeks, and 6 months). Extended HIV follow-up (e.g., for 12 months) is recommended for HCP who become infected with HCV following exposure to a source coinfected with HIV and HCV. Whether extended follow-up is indicated in other circumstances (e.g., exposure to a source coinfected with HIV and HCV in the absence of HCV seroconversion or for exposed persons with a medical history suggesting an impaired ability to develop an antibody response to acute infection) is unclear. Although rare instances of delayed HIV seroconversion have been reported (*167,168*), the infrequency of this occurrence does not warrant adding to the anxiety level of the exposed persons by routinely extending the duration of postexposure follow-up. However, this recommendation should not preclude a decision to extend follow-up in an individual situation based on the clinical judgement of the exposed person's health-care provider. HIV testing should be performed on any exposed person who has an illness that is compatible with an acute retroviral syndrome, regardless of the interval since exposure. When HIV infection is identified, the person should be referred to a specialist knowledgeable in the area of HIV treatment and counseling for medical management.

HIV-antibody testing with EIA should be used to monitor for seroconversion. The routine use of direct virus assays (e.g., HIV p24 antigen EIA or tests for HIV RNA) to detect infection in exposed HCP generally is not recommended (*169*). The high rate of false-positive results of these tests in this setting could lead to unnecessary anxiety and/or treatment (*170,171*). Despite the ability of direct virus assays to detect HIV infection a few days earlier than EIA, the infrequency of occupational seroconversion and increased costs of these tests do not warrant their routine use in this setting.

- HIV-antibody testing should be performed for at least 6 months postexposure.
- Direct virus assays for routine follow-up of HCP are not recommended.
- HIV testing should be performed on any exposed person who has an illness compatible with an acute retroviral syndrome.

Monitoring and Management of PEP Toxicity. If PEP is used, HCP should be monitored for drug toxicity by testing at baseline and again 2 weeks after starting PEP. The scope of testing should be based on medical conditions in the exposed person and the toxicity of drugs included in the PEP regimen. Minimally, lab monitoring for toxicity should include a complete blood count and renal and hepatic function tests. Monitoring for evidence of hyperglycemia should be included for HCP whose regimens include any PI; if the exposed person is receiving IDV, monitoring for crystalluria, hematuria, hemolytic anemia, and hepatitis also should be included. If toxicity is noted, modification of the regimen should be considered after expert consultation; further diagnostic studies may be indicated.

Exposed HCP who choose to take PEP should be advised of the importance of completing the prescribed regimen. Information should be provided to HCP about potential drug interactions and the drugs that should not be taken with PEP, the side effects of the drugs that have been prescribed, measures to minimize these effects, and the methods of clinical monitoring for toxicity during the follow-up period. HCP should be advised that the evaluation of certain symptoms should not be delayed (e.g., rash, fever, back or abdominal pain, pain on urination or blood in the urine, or symptoms of hyperglycemia [increased thirst and/or frequent urination]).

HCP who fail to complete the recommended regimen often do so because of the side effects they experience (e.g., nausea and diarrhea). These symptoms often can be managed with antimotility and antiemetic agents or other medications that target the specific symptoms without changing the regimen. In other situations, modifying the dose interval (i.e., administering a lower dose of drug more frequently throughout the day, as recommended by the manufacturer), might facilitate adherence to the regimen. Serious adverse events should be reported to FDA's MedWatch Program.

Counseling and Education. Although HIV infection following an occupational exposure occurs infrequently, the emotional effect of an exposure often is substantial (*172--174*). In addition, HCP are given seemingly conflicting information. Although HCP are told that a low risk exists for HIV transmission, a 4-week regimen of PEP might be recommended, and they are asked to commit to behavioral measures (e.g., sexual abstinence or condom use) to prevent secondary transmission, all of which influence their lives for several weeks to months (*172*). Therefore, access to persons who are knowledgeable about occupational HIV transmission and who can deal with the many concerns an HIV exposure might generate for the exposed person is an important element of postexposure management. HIV-exposed HCP should be advised to use the following measures to prevent secondary transmission during the follow-up period, especially the first 6--12 weeks after the exposure when most HIV-infected persons are expected to seroconvert: exercise sexual abstinence or use condoms to prevent sexual transmission and to avoid pregnancy; and refrain from donating blood, plasma, organs, tissue, or semen. If an exposed woman is breast feeding, she should be counseled about the risk of HIV transmission through breast milk, and discontinuation of breast feeding should be considered, especially for high-risk exposures. Additionally, NRTIs are known to pass into breast milk, as is NVP; whether this also is true for the other approved antiretroviral drugs is unknown.

The patient-care responsibilities of an exposed person do not need to be modified, based solely on an HIV exposure, to prevent transmission to patients. If HIV seroconversion is detected, the person should be evaluated according to published recommendations for infected HCP (*175*).

Exposed HCP should be advised to seek medical evaluation for any acute illness that occurs during the follow-up period. Such an illness, particularly if characterized by fever, rash, myalgia, fatigue, malaise, or lymphadenopathy, might be indicative of acute HIV infection but also might be indicative of a drug reaction or another medical condition.

For exposures for which PEP is considered appropriate, HCP should be informed that a) knowledge about the efficacy of drugs used for PEP is limited; b) experts recommend combination drug regimens because of increased potency and concerns about drug-resistant virus; c) data regarding toxicity of antiretroviral drugs in persons without HIV infection or in pregnant women are limited; d) although the short-term toxicity of antiretroviral drugs is usually limited, serious adverse events have occurred in persons taking PEP; and e) any or all drugs for PEP may be declined or stopped by the exposed person. HCP who experience HIV occupational exposures for which PEP is not recommended should be informed that the potential side effects and toxicity of taking PEP outweigh the negligible risk of transmission posed by the type of exposure.

Guidelines for counseling and educating HCP with HIV exposure include

- Exposed HCP should be advised to use precautions to prevent secondary transmission during the follow-up period.
- For exposures for which PEP is prescribed, HCP should be informed about possible drug toxicities and the need for monitoring, and possible drug interactions.

Occupational Exposure Management Resources

Several resources are available that provide guidance to HCP regarding the management of occupational exposures. These resources include PEPline; the Needlestick! website; the Hepatitis Hotline; CDC (receives reports of occupationally acquired HIV infections and failures of PEP); the HIV Antiretroviral Pregnancy Registry; FDA (receives reports of unusual or severe toxicity to antiretroviral agents); and the HIV/AIDS Treatment Information Service (Box 5).

*This interagency working group comprised representatives of CDC, the Food and Drug Administration (FDA), the Health Resources and Services Administration, and the National Institutes of Health. Information included in these recommendations may not represent FDA approval or approved labeling for the particular product or indications in question. Specifically, the terms "safe" and "effective" may not be synonymous with the FDA-defined legal standards for product approval.

References

1. CDC. NIOSH alert: preventing needlestick injuries in health care settings. Cincinnati, OH: Department of Health and Human Services, CDC, 1999; DHHS publication no. (NIOSH)2000-108.
2. Department of Labor, Occupational Safety and Health Administration. 29 CFR Part 1910.1030. Occupational exposure to bloodborne pathogens; final rule. Federal Register 1991; 56:64004--182.
3. CDC. Public Health Service statement on management of occupational exposure to human immunodeficiency virus, including considerations regarding zidovudine postexposure use. MMWR 1990;39(No. RR-1).
4. CDC. Update: provisional Public Health Service recommendations for chemoprophylaxis after occupational exposure to HIV. MMWR 1996;45:468--72.
5. CDC. Public Health Service guidelines for the management of health-care worker exposures to HIV and recommendations for postexposure prophylaxis. MMWR 1998;47(No. RR-7).
6. Panlilio AL, Cardo DM, Campbell S, Srivastava P, NaSH Surveillance Group. Experience of health care workers taking antiretroviral agents as postexposure prophylaxis for occupational exposure to HIV [Abstract 489]. In: Proceedings of the 1999 National HIV Prevention Conference. Atlanta, GA, 1999.
7. Wang SA, Panlilio AL, Doi PA, et al. Experience of healthcare workers taking postexposure prophylaxis after occupational HIV exposures: findings of the HIV postexposure prophylaxis registry. Infect Control Hosp Epidemiol 2000;21:780--5.
8. Puro V, Ippolito G, Italian Registry PEP. Antiretroviral post-exposure prophylaxis [Abstract 515]. In: Proceedings of the 1999 National HIV Prevention Conference. Atlanta, GA, 1999.
9. Parkin JM, Murphy M, Anderson J, El-Gadi S, Forster G, Pinching AJ. Tolerability and side-effects of post-exposure prophylaxis for HIV infection [Letter]. Lancet 2000;355:722--3.
10. Jochimsen EM, Srivastava PU, Campbell SR, Cardo DM, NaSH Surveillance Group. Postexposure prophylaxis (PEP) use among health care workers (HCWs) after occupational exposures to blood [Abstract W6-F]. In: Keynote addresses and abstracts of the 4th ICOH International Conference on Occupational Health for Health Care Workers. Montreal, Canada, 1999.
11. Critchley SE, Srivastava PU, Campbell SR, Cardo DM, NaSH Surveillance Group. Postexposure prophylaxis use among healthcare workers who were exposed to HIV-negative source persons [Abstract P-S2-64]. In: Program and Abstracts of the 4th Decennial International Conference on Nosocomial and Healthcare-Associated Infections. Atlanta, GA: CDC in conjunction with the 10th Annual Meeting of SHEA, 2000:126.
12. CDC. Hepatitis B virus: a comprehensive strategy for eliminating transmission in the United States through universal childhood vaccination: recommendations of the Immunization Practices Advisory Committee (ACIP). MMWR 1991;40(No. RR-13).
13. CDC. Recommendations for the prevention and control of hepatitis C virus (HCV) infection and HCV-related chronic disease. MMWR 1998;47(No. RR-19).
14. CDC. Management of possible sexual, injecting-drug--use, or other nonoccupational exposure to HIV, including considerations related to antiretroviral therapy: Public Health Service statement. MMWR 1998;47(no. RR-17).
15. CDC. Recommendations of the U.S. Public Health Service Task Force on the use of zidovudine to reduce perinatal transmission of human immunodeficiency virus. MMWR 1994;43(No. RR-11).
16. CDC. Recommendations for prevention of HIV transmission in health-care settings. MMWR 1987;36(suppl no. 2S).
17. CDC. Update: universal precautions for prevention of transmission of human immunodeficiency virus, hepatitis B virus, and other bloodborne pathogens in health-care settings. MMWR 1988;37:377--82,387--8.
18. Shapiro CN, McCaig LF, Gensheimer KF, et al. Hepatitis B virus transmission between children in day care. Pediatr Infect Dis J 1989;8:870--5.
19. Richman KM, Rickman LS. The potential for transmission of human immunodeficiency virus through human bites. J Acquir Immune Defic Syndr 1993;6:402--6.

20. Vidmar L, Poljak M, Tomazic J, Seme K, Klavs I. Transmission of HIV-1 by human bite [Letter]. Lancet 1996;347:1762--3.

21. CDC. Immunization of health-care workers: recommendations of the Advisory Committee on Immunization Practices (ACIP) and the Hospital Infection Control Practices Advisory Committee (HICPAC). MMWR 1997;46(No. RR-18).

22. Chiarello LA, Gerberding JL. Human immunodeficiency virus in health care settings. In: Mandell GL, Bennett JE, Dolin R, eds. Mandell, Douglas, and Bennett's principles and practice of infectious diseases. 5th ed. Philadelphia, PA: Churchill Livingstone, 2000:3052--66.

23. Cardo DM, Smith DK, Bell DM. Postexposure Management. In: Dolin R, Masur H, Saag MS, eds. AIDS Therapy. New York, NY: Churchill Livingstone, 1999:236--47.

24. Beltrami EM, Williams IT, Shapiro CN, Chamberland ME. Risk and management of blood-borne infections in health care workers. Clin Microbiol Rev 2000;13:385--407.

25. Mast EE, Alter MJ. Prevention of hepatitis B virus infection among health-care workers. In: Ellis RW, ed. Hepatitis B vaccines in clinical practice. New York, NY: Marcel Dekker, 1993:295--307.

26. Werner BG, Grady GF. Accidental hepatitis-B-surface-antigen-positive inoculations: use of e antigen to estimate infectivity. Ann Intern Med 1982;97:367--9.

27. Garibaldi RA, Hatch FE, Bisno AL, Hatch MH, Gregg MB. Nonparenteral serum hepatitis: report of an outbreak. JAMA 1972;220:963--6.

28. Rosenberg JL, Jones DP, Lipitz LR, Kirsner JB. Viral hepatitis: an occupational hazard to surgeons. JAMA 1973;223:395--400.

29. Callender ME, White YS, Williams R. Hepatitis B virus infection in medical and health care personnel. Br Med J 1982;284:324--6.

30. Chaudhuri AKR, Follett EAC. Hepatitis B virus infection in medical and health care personnel [Letter]. Br Med J 1982;284:1408.

31. Bond WW, Favero MS, Petersen NJ, Gravelle CR, Ebert JW, Maynard JE. Survival of hepatitis B virus after drying and storage for one week [Letter]. Lancet 1981;1:550--1.

32. Francis DP, Favero MS, Maynard JE. Transmission of hepatitis B virus. Semin Liver Dis 1981;1:27--32.

33. Favero MS, Maynard JE, Petersen NJ, et al. HepatitisB antigen on environmental surfaces [Letter]. Lancet 1973;2:1455.

34. Lauer JL, VanDrunen NA, Washburn JW, Balfour HH Jr. Transmission of hepatitis B virus in clinical laboratory areas. J Infect Dis 1979;140:513--6.

35. Hennekens CH. Hemodialysis-associated hepatitis: an outbreak among hospital personnel. JAMA 1973;225:407--8.

36. Garibaldi RA, Forrest JN, Bryan JA, Hanson BF, Dismukes WE. Hemodialysis-associated hepatitis. JAMA 1973;225:384--9.

37. Snydman DR, Bryan JA, Macon EJ, Gregg MB. Hemodialysis-associated hepatitis: a report of an epidemic with further evidence on mechanisms of transmission. Am J Epidemiol 1976;104:563--70.

38. Bond WW, Petersen NJ, Favero MS. Viral hepatitis B: aspects of environmental control. Health Lab Sci 1977;14:235--52.

39. Segal HE, Llewellyn CH, Irwin G, Bancroft WH, Boe GP, Balaban DJ. Hepatitis B antigen and antibody in the U.S. Army: prevalence in health care personnel. Am J Pub Health 1976;55:667--71.

40. Denes AE, Smith JL, Maynard JE, Doto IL, Berquist KR, Finkel AJ. Hepatitis B infection in physicians: results of a nationwide seroepidemiologic survey. JAMA 1978;239:210--2.

41. Dienstag JL, Ryan DM. Occupational exposure to hepatitis B virus in hospital personnel: infection or immunization? Am J Epidemiol 1982;115:26--39.

42. West DJ. The risk of hepatitis B infection among health professionals in the United States: a review. Am J Med Sci 1984;287:26--33.

43. CDC. Recommendation of the Immunization Practices Advisory Committee (ACIP) inactivated hepatitis B virus vaccine. MMWR 1982;31:317--28.

44. Beasley RP, Hwang L-Y, Lee G C-Y, et al. Prevention of perinatally transmitted hepatitis B virus infections with hepatitis B immune globulin and hepatitis B vaccine. Lancet 1983;2:1099--102.

45. Stevens CE, Toy PT, Tong MJ, et al. Perinatal hepatitis B virus transmission in the United States: prevention by passive-active immunization. JAMA 1985;253:1740--5.

46. Beasley RP, Hwang L-Y, Stevens CE, et al. Efficacy of hepatitis B immune globulin for prevention of perinatal transmission of the hepatitis B virus carrier state: final report of a randomized double-blind, placebo-controlled trial. Hepatology 1983;3:135--41.

47. Grady GF, Lee VA, Prince AM, et al. Hepatitis B immune globulin for accidental exposures among medical personnel: final report of a multicenter controlled trial. J Infect Dis 1978;138:625--38.

48. Seeff LB, Zimmerman HJ, Wright EC, et al. A randomized, double blind controlled trial of the efficacy of immune serum globulin for the prevention of post-transfusion hepatitis: a Veterans Administration cooperative study. Gastroenterology 1977;72:111--21.

49. Prince AM, Szmuness W, Mann MK, et al. Hepatitis B "immune" globulin: effectiveness in prevention of dialysis-associated hepatitis. N Engl J Med 1975;293:1063--7.

50. Greenberg DP. Pediatric experience with recombinant hepatitis B vaccines and relevant safety and immunogenicity studies. Pediatr Inf Dis J 1993;12:438--45.

51. Szmuness W, Stevens CE, Harley EJ, et al. Hepatitis B vaccine: demonstration of efficacy in a controlled clinical trial in a high-risk population in the United States. N Engl J Med 1980;303:833--41.

52. Francis DP, Hadler SC, Thompson SE, et al. The prevention of hepatitis B with vaccine: report of the Centers for Disease Control multi-center efficacy trial among homosexual men. Ann Intern Med 1982;97:362--6.

53. Stevens CE, Alter HJ, Taylor PE, et al. Hepatitis B vaccine in patients receiving hemodialysis: immunogenicity and efficacy. N Engl J Med 1984;311:496--501.

54. André FE. Summary of safety and efficacy data on a yeast-derived hepatitis B vaccine. Am J Med 1989;87(suppl 3A):14S--20S.

55. Zajac BA, West DJ, McAleer WJ, Scolnick EM. Overview of clinical studies with hepatitis B vaccine made by recombinant DNA. J Infect 1986;13(suppl A):39--45.

56. Wise RP, Kiminyo KP, Salive ME. Hair loss after routine immunizations. JAMA 1997;278:1176--8.

57. Shaw FE, Graham DJ, Guess HA, et al. Postmarketing surveillance for neurologic adverse events reported after hepatitis B vaccination: experience of the first three years. Am J Epidemiol 1988;127:337--52.

58. Chen D-S. Control of hepatitis B in Asia: mass immunization program in Taiwan. In: Hollinger FB, Lemon SM, Margolis HS, eds. Viral hepatitis and liver disease. Baltimore, MD: Williams and Wilkins, 1991:716--9.

59. Niu MT, Rhodes P, Salive M, et al. Comparative safety of two recombinant hepatitis B vaccines in children: data from the Vaccine Adverse Event Reporting System (VAERS) and Vaccine Safety Datalink (VSD). J Clin Epidemiol 1998;51:503--10.

60. Ribera EF, Dutka AJ. Polyneuropathy associated with administration of hepatitis B vaccine [Letter]. N Engl J Med 1983;309:614--5.

61. Tuohy PG. Guillain-Barré syndrome following immunisation with synthetic hepatitis B vaccine [Letter]. N Z Med J 1989;102:114--5.

62. Herroelen L, de Keyser J, Ebinger G. Central-nervous-system demyelination after immunisation with recombinant hepatitis B vaccine. Lancet 1991;338:1174--5.

63. Gross K, Combe C, Krüger K, Schattenkirchner M. Arthritis after hepatitis B vaccination: report of three cases. Scand J Rheumatol 1995;24:50--2.

64. Pope JE, Stevens A, Howson W, Bell DA. The development of rheumatoid arthritis after recombinant hepatitis B vaccination. J Rheumatol 1998;25:1687--93.

65. Hassan W, Oldham R. Reiter's syndrome and reactive arthritis in health care workers after vaccination. Br Med J 1994;309:94.

66. Grotto I, Mandel Y, Ephros M, Ashkenazi I, Shemer J. Major adverse reactions to yeast-derived hepatitis B vaccines---a review. Vaccine 1998;16:329--34.

67. Confavreux C, Suissa S, Saddier P, Bourdès V, Vukusic S, Vaccines in Multiple Sclerosis Study Group. Vaccinations and the risk of relapse in multiple sclerosis. N Engl J Med 2001;344:319--26.

68. Ascherio A, Zhang SM, Hernán MA, et al. Hepatitis B vaccination and the risk of multiple sclerosis. N Engl J Med 2001;344:327--32.

69. Halsey NA, Duclos P, Van Damme P, Margolis H. Hepatitis B vaccine and central nervous system demyelinating diseases. Viral Hepatitis Prevention Board. Pediatr Infect Dis J 1999;18:23--4.

70. CDC. Safety of therapeutic immune globulin preparations with respect to transmission of human T-lymphotropic virus type III/lymphadenopathy-associated virus infection. MMWR 1986;35:231--3.

71. CDC. Outbreak of hepatitis C associated with intravenous immunoglobulin administration---United States, October 1993--June 1994, MMWR 1994;43:505--9.

72. Ellis EF, Henney CS. Adverse reactions following administration of human gamma globulin. J Allerg 1969;43:45--54.

73. Alter MJ. The epidemiology of acute and chronic hepatitis C. Clin Liver Dis 1997;1:559--68.

74. Lanphear BP, Linnemann CC Jr., Cannon CG, DeRonde MM, Pendy L, Kerley LM. Hepatitis C virus infection in healthcare workers: risk of exposure and infection. Infect Control Hosp Epidemiol 1994;15:745--50.

75. Puro V, Petrosillo N, Ippolito G, Italian Study Group on Occupational Risk of HIV and Other Bloodborne Infections. Risk of hepatitis C seroconversion after occupational exposure in health care workers. Am J Infect Control 1995;23:273--7.

76. Mitsui T, Iwano K, Masuko K, et al. Hepatitis C virus infection in medical personnel after needlestick accident. Hepatology 1992;16:1109--14.

77. Sartori M, La Terra G, Aglietta M, Manzin A, Navino C, Verzetti G. Transmission of hepatitis C via blood splash into conjunctiva [Letter]. Scand J Infect Dis 1993;25:270--1.

78. Ippolito G, Puro V, Petrosillo N, et al. Simultaneous infection with HIV and hepatitis C virus following occupational conjunctival blood exposure [Letter]. JAMA 1998;280:28.

79. Davis GL, Lau J Y-N, Urdea MS, et al. Quantitative detection of hepatitis C virus RNA with a solid-phase signal amplification method: definition of optimal conditions for specimen collection and clinical application in interferon-treated patients. Hepatology 1994;19:1337--41.

80. Polish LB, Tong MJ, Co RL, Coleman PJ, Alter MJ. Risk factors for hepatitis C virus infection among health care personnel in a community hospital. Am J Infect Control 1993;21:196--200.

81. Niu MT, Coleman PJ, Alter MJ. Multicenter study of hepatitis C virus infection in chronic hemodialysis patients and hemodialysis center staff members. Am J Kidney Dis 1993;22:568--73.

82. Hardy NM, Sandroni S, Danielson S, Wilson WJ. Antibody to hepatitis C virus increases with time on hemodialysis. Clin Nephrol 1992;38:44--8.

83. Niu MT, Alter MJ, Kristensen C, Margolis HS. Outbreak of hemodialysis-associated non-A, non-B hepatitis and correlation with antibody to hepatitis C virus. Am J Kidney Dis 1992;19:345--52.

84. Favero MS, Alter MJ. The reemergence of hepatitis B virus infection in hemodialysis centers. Semin Dial 1996;9:373--4.

85. Knodell RG, Conrad ME, Ginsberg AL, Bell CJ, Flannery EPR. Efficacy of prophylactic gamma-globulin in preventing non-A, non-B post-transfusion hepatitis. Lancet 1976;1:557--61.

86. Sanchez-Quijano A, Pineda JA, Lissen E, et al. Prevention of post-transfusion non-A, non-B hepatitis by non-specific immunoglobulin in heart surgery patients. Lancet 1988;1:1245--9.

87. Krawczynski K, Alter MJ, Tankersley DL, et al. Effect of immune globulin on the prevention of experimental hepatitis C virus infection. J Infect Dis 1996;173:822--8.

88. Alter MJ. Occupational exposure to hepatitis C virus: a dilemma. Infect Control Hosp Epidemiol 1994;15:742--4.

89. Peters M, Davis GL, Dooley JS, Hoofnagle JH. The interferon system in acute and chronic viral hepatitis. Progress in Liver Diseases 1986;8:453--67.

90. Fried MW, Hoofnagle JH. Therapy of hepatitis C. Semin Liver Dis 1995;15:82--91.

91. Vogel W, Graziadei I, Umlauft F, et al. High-dose interferon-a_{2b} treatment prevents chronicity in acute hepatitis C: a pilot study. Dig Dis Sci 1996;41(suppl 12):81S--85S.

92. Quin JW. Interferon therapy for acute hepatitis C viral infection---a review by meta-analysis. Aust N Z J Med 1997;27:611--7.

93. Seeff LB, Hollinger FB, Alter HJ, et al. Long-term mortality and morbidity of transfusion-associated non-A, non-B, and type C hepatitis: a National Heart, Lung, and Blood Institute collaborative study. Hepatology 2001;33:455--63.

94. Bell DM. Occupational risk of human immunodeficiency virus infection in healthcare workers: an overview. Am J Med 1997;102(suppl 5B):9--15.

95. Ippolito G, Puro V, De Carli G, Italian Study Group on Occupational Risk of HIV Infection. The risk of occupational human immunodeficiency virus in health care workers. Arch Int Med 1993;153:1451--8.

96. CDC. Update: human immunodeficiency virus infections in health-care workers exposed to blood of infected patients. MMWR 1987;36:285--9.

97. Fahey BJ, Koziol DE, Banks SM, Henderson DK. Frequency of nonparenteral occupational exposures to blood and body fluids before and after universal precautions training. Am J Med 1991;90:145--53.

98. Henderson DK, Fahey BJ, Willy M, et al. Risk for occupational transmission of human immunodeficiency virus type 1 (HIV-1) associated with clinical exposures: a prospective evaluation. Ann Intern Med 1990;113:740--6.

99. CDC. HIV/AIDS Surveillance Report. Atlanta, GA: Department of Health and Human Services, CDC, 2000:24. (vol 12, no. 1).

100. Cardo DM, Culver DH, Ciesielski CA, et al. A case-control study of HIV seroconversion in health care workers after percutaneous exposure. N Engl J Med 1997;337:1485--90.

101. Mast ST, Woolwine JD, Gerberding JL. Efficacy of gloves in reducing blood volumes transferred during simulated needlestick injury. J Infect Dis 1993;168:1589--92.

102. Pinto LA, Landay AL, Berzofsky JA, Kessler HA, Shearer GM. Immune response to human immunodeficiency virus (HIV) in healthcare workers occupationally exposed to HIV-contaminated blood. Am J Med 1997;102(suppl 5B):21--4.

103. Clerici M, Giorgi JV, Chou C-C, et al. Cell-mediated immune response to human immunodeficiency virus (HIV) type 1 in seronegative homosexual men with recent sexual exposure to HIV-1. J Infect Dis 1992;165:1012--9.

104. Ranki A, Mattinen S, Yarchoan R, et al. T-cell response towards HIV in infected individuals with and without zidovudine therapy, and in HIV-exposed sexual partners. AIDS 1989;3:63--9.

105. Cheynier R, Langlade-Demoyen P, Marescot M-R, et al. Cytotoxic T lymphocyte responses in the peripheral blood of children born to human immunodeficiency virus-1-infected mothers. Eur J Immunol 1992;22:2211--7.

106. Kelker HC, Seidlin M, Vogler M, Valentine FT. Lymphocytes from some long-term seronegative heterosexual partners of HIV-infected individuals proliferate in response to HIV antigens. AIDS Res Hum Retroviruses 1992;8:1355--9.

107. Langlade-Demoyen P, Ngo-Giang-Huong N, Ferchal F, Oksenhendler E. Human immunodeficiency virus (HIV) nef-specific cytotoxic T lymphocytes in noninfected heterosexual contact of HIV-infected patients. J Clin Invest 1994;93:1293--7.

108. Rowland-Jones S, Sutton J, Ariyoshi K, et al. HIV-specific cytotoxic T-cells in HIV-exposed but uninfected Gambian women. Nat Med 1995;1:59--64.

109. D'Amico R, Pinto LA, Meyer P, et al. Effect of zidovudine postexposure prophylaxis on the development of HIV-specific cytotoxic T-lymphocyte responses in HIV-exposed healthcare workers. Infect Control Hosp Epidemiol 1999;20:428--30.

110. Spira AI, Marx PA, Patterson BK, et al. Cellular targets of infection and route of viral dissemination after an intravaginal inoculation of simian immunodeficiency virus into rhesus macaques. J Exp Med 1996;183:215--25.

111. McClure HM, Anderson DC, Ansari AA, Fultz PN, Klumpp SA, Schinazi RF. Nonhuman primate models for evaluation of AIDS therapy. In: AIDS: anti-HIV agents, therapies and vaccines. Ann N Y Acad Sci 1990;616:287--98.

112. Böttiger D, Johansson N-G, Samuelsson B, et al. Prevention of simian immunodeficiency virus, SIV_{sm}, or HIV-2 infection in cynomolgus monkeys by pre- and postexposure administration of BEA-005. AIDS 1997;11:157--62.

113. Otten RA, Smith DK, Adams DR, et al. Efficacy of postexposure prophylaxis after intravaginal exposure of pig-tailed macaques to a human-derived retrovirus (human immunodeficiency virus type 2). J Virol 2000;74:9771--5.

114. Sinet M, Desforges B, Launay O, Colin J-N, Pocidalo J-J. Factors influencing zidovudine efficacy when administered at early stages of Friend virus infection in mice. Antiviral Res 1991;16:163--71.

115. Ruprecht RM, Bronson R. Chemoprevention of retroviral infection: success is determined by virus inoculum strength and cellular immunity. DNA Cell Biol 1994;13:59--66.

116. Fazely F, Haseltine WA, Rodger RF, Ruprecht RM. Postexposure chemoprophylaxis with ZDV or ZDV combined with interferon-a: failure after inoculating rhesus monkeys with a high dose of SIV. J Acquir Immune Defic Syndr 1991;4:1093--7.

117. Böttiger D, Oberg B. Influence of the infectious dose of SIV on the acute infection in cynomolgus monkeys and on the effect of treatment with 3'-fluorothymidine [Abstract no. 81]. In: Symposium on Nonhuman Primate Models for AIDS. Seattle, WA, 1991.

118. Martin LN, Murphey-Corb M, Soike KF, Davison-Fairburn B, Baskin GB. Effects of initiation of 3'-azido,3'-deoxythymidine (zidovudine) treatment at different times after infection of rhesus monkeys with simian immunodeficiency virus. J Infect Dis 1993;168:825--35.

119. Shih C-C, Kaneshima H, Rabin L, et al. Postexposure prophylaxis with zidovudine suppresses human immunodeficiency virus type 1 infection in SCID-hu mice in a time-dependent manner. J Infect Dis 1991;163:625--7.

120. Mathes LE, Polas PJ, Hayes KA, Swenson CL, Johnson S, Kociba GJ. Pre- and postexposure chemoprophylaxis: evidence that 3'-azido-3'dideoxythymidine inhibits feline leukemia virus disease by a drug-induced vaccine response. Antimicrob Agents Chemother 1992;36:2715--21.

121. Tavares L, Roneker C, Johnston K, Lehrman SN, de Noronha F. 3'-azido-3'-deoxythymidine in feline leukemia virus-infected cats: a model for therapy and prophylaxis of AIDS. Cancer Res 1987;47:3190--4.

122. Tsai C-C, Follis KE, Sabo A, et al. Prevention of SIV infection in macaques by (R)-9-(2-phosphonylmethoxypropyl) adenine. Science 1995;270:1197--9.

123. Tsai C-C, Emau P, Follis KE, et al. Effectiveness of postinoculation (R)-9-(2-phosphonylmethoxypropyl) adenine treatment for prevention of persistent simian immunodeficiency virus SIV_{mne} infection depends critically on timing of initiation and duration of treatment. J Virol 1998;72:4265--73.

124. Le Grand R, Vaslin B, Larghero J, et al. Post-exposure prophylaxis with highly active antiretroviral therapy could not protect macaques from infection with SIV/HIV chimera. AIDS 2000;14:1864--6.

125. LaFon SW, Mooney BD, McMullen JP, et al. A double-blind, placebo-controlled study of the safety and efficacy of retrovir® (zidovudine, ZDV) as a chemoprophylactic agent in health care workers exposed to HIV [Abstract 489]. In: Program and abstracts of the 30th Interscience Conference on Antimicrobial Agents and Chemotherapy. Atlanta, GA: American Society for Microbiology, 1990:167.

126. Connor EM, Sperling RS, Gelber R, et al. Reduction of maternal-infant transmission of human immunodeficiency virus type 1 with zidovudine treatment. N Engl J Med 1994;331:1173--80.

127. Sperling RS, Shapiro DE, Coombs RW, et al. Maternal viral load, zidovudine treatment, and the risk of transmission of human immunodeficiency virus type 1 from mother to infant. N Engl J Med 1996;335:1621--9.

128. Shaffer N, Chuachoowong R, Mock PA, et al. Short-course zidovudine for perinatal HIV-1 transmission in Bangkok, Thailand: a randomised controlled trial. Lancet 1999;353: 773--80.

129. Saba J, PETRA Trial Study Team. Interim analysis of early efficacy of three short ZDV/3TC combination regimens to prevent mother-to-child transmission of HIV-1: the PETRA trial [Abstract S-7]. In: Program and abstracts of the 6th Conference on Retroviruses and Opportunistic Infections. Chicago, IL: Foundation for Retrovirology and Human Health in scientific collaboration with the National Institute of Allergy and Infectious Diseases and CDC, 1999.

130. Wade NA, Birkhead GS, Warren BL, et al. Abbreviated regimens of zidovudine prophylaxis and perinatal transmission of the human immunodeficiency virus. N Engl J Med 1998;339:1409--14.

131. Musoke P, Guay LA, Bagenda D, et al. A phase I/II study of the safety and pharmacokinetics of nevirapine in HIV-1-infected pregnant Ugandan women and their neonates (HIVNET 006). AIDS 1999;13:479--86.

132. Guay LA, Musoke P, Fleming T, et al. Intrapartum and neonatal single-dose nevirapine compared with zidovudine for prevention of mother-to-child transmission of HIV-1 in Kampala, Uganda: HIVNET 012 randomised trial. Lancet 1999;354:795--802.

133. Jochimsen EM. Failures of zidovudine postexposure prophylaxis. Am J Med 1997;102(suppl 5B):52--5.

134. Pratt RD, Shapiro JF, McKinney N, Kwok S, Spector SA. Virologic characterization of primary human immunodeficiency virus type 1 infection in a health care worker following needlestick injury. J Infect Dis 1995;172:851--4.

135. Lot F, Abiteboul D. Infections professionnelles par le V.I.H. en France chez le personnel de santé--le point au 30 juin 1995. Bulletin Épidémiologique Hebdomadaire 1995;44:193--4.

136. Weisburd G, Biglione J, Arbulu MM, Terrazzino JC, Pesiri A. HIV seroconversion after a work place accident and treated with zidovudine [Abstract Pub.C.1141]. In: Abstracts of the XI International Conference on AIDS. Vancouver, British Columbia, Canada, 1996:460.

137. Perdue B, Wolderufael D, Mellors J, Quinn T, Margolick J. HIV-1 transmission by a needlestick injury despite rapid initiation of four-drug postexposure prophylaxis [Abstract 210]. In: Program and abstracts of the 6th Conference on Retroviruses and Opportunistic Infections. Chicago, IL: Foundation for Retrovirology and Human Health in scientific collaboration with the National Institute of Allergy and Infectious Diseases and CDC, 1999:107.

138. Lot F, Abiteboul D. Occupational HIV infection in France [Abstract WP-25]. In: Keynote addresses and abstracts of the 4th ICOH International Conference on Occupational Health for Health Care Workers. Montreal, Canada, 1999.

139. Beltrami EM, Luo C-C, Dela Torre N, Cardo DM. HIV transmission after an occupational exposure despite postexposure prophylaxis with a combination drug regimen [Abstract P-S2-62]. In: Program and abstracts of the 4th Decennial International Conference on Nosocomial and Healthcare-Associated Infections in conjunction with the 10th Annual Meeting of SHEA. Atlanta, GA: CDC, 2000:125--6.

140. Panel on Clinical Practices for Treatment of HIV Infection. Guidelines for the use of antiretroviral agents in HIV-infected adults and adolescents. Available at <http://hivatis.org/trtgdlns.html>. Accessed May 9, 2001.

141. Manion DJ, Hirsch MS. Combination chemotherapy for human immunodeficiency virus-1. Am J Med 1997;102(suppl 5B):76--80.

142. Lafeuillade A, Poggi C, Tamalet C, Profizi N, Tourres C, Costes O. Effects of a combination of zidovudine, didanosine, and lamivudine on primary human immunodeficiency virus type 1 infection. J Infect Dis 1997;175:1051--5.

143. Beltrami EM, Cheingsong R, Respess R, Cardo DM. Antiretroviral drug resistance in HIV-infected source patients for occupational exposures to healthcare workers [Abstract P-S2-70]. In: Program and Abstracts of the 4th Decennial International Conference on Nosocomial and Healthcare-Associated Infections. Atlanta, GA: CDC, 2000:128.

144. Struble KA, Pratt RD, Gitterman SR. Toxicity of antiretroviral agents. Am J Med 1997;102(suppl 5B):65--7.

145. Food and Drug Administration. Protease inhibitors may increase blood glucose in HIV patients. FDA Medical Bulletin 1997;27(2).

146. Dever LL, Oruwari PA, O'Donovan CA, Eng RHK. Hyperglycemia associated with protease inhibitors in HIV-infected patients [Abstract LB-4]. In: Abstracts of the 37th Interscience Conference on Antimicrobial Agents and Chemotherapy. Toronto, Ontario, Canada: American Society for Microbiology, 1997.

147. Dubé MP, Johnson DL, Currier JS, Leedom JM. Protease inhibitor-associated hyperglycaemia [Letter]. Lancet 1997;350:713--4.

148. Abramowicz M, ed. New drugs for HIV infection. The Medical Letter on Drugs and Therapeutics 1996;38:35--7.

149. Martin JN, Roland ME, Bamberger JD, et al. Postexposure prophylaxis after sexual or drug use exposure to HIV: final results from the San Francisco Post-Exposure Prevention (PEP) Project [Abstract 196]. In: Program and abstracts of the 7th Conference on Retroviruses and Opportunistic Infections. San Francisco, CA: Foundation for Retrovirology and Human Health in scientific collaboration with the National Institute of Allergy and Infectious Diseases and CDC, 2000:112.

150. Steger KA, Swotinsky R, Snyder S, Craven DE. Recent experience with post-exposure prophylaxis (PEP) with combination antiretrovirals for occupational exposure (OE) to HIV [Abstract 480]. In: Program and abstracts of the 35th annual meeting of the Infectious Diseases Society of America. Alexandria, VA: Infectious Diseases Society of America, 1997:161.

151. Henry K, Acosta EP, Jochimsen E. Hepatotoxicity and rash associated with zidovudine and zalcitabine chemoprophylaxis [Letter]. Ann Intern Med 1996;124:855.

152. Johnson S, Baraboutis JG; Sha BE, Proia LA, Kessler HA. Adverse effects associated with use of nevirapine in HIV postexposure prophylaxis for 2 health care workers [Letters]. JAMA 2000;284:2722--3.

153. CDC. Serious adverse events attributed to nevirapine regimens for postexposure prophylaxis after HIV exposures---worldwide, 1997--2000. MMWR 2001;49:1153--6.

154. Hirsch MS, Brun-Vézinet F, D'Aquila RT, et al. Antiretroviral drug resistance testing in adult HIV-1 infection: recommendations of an international AIDS Society---USA panel. JAMA 2000;283:2417--26.

155. Tack PC, Bremer JW, Harris AA, Landay AL, Kessler HA. Genotypic analysis of HIV-1 isolates to identify antiretroviral resistance mutations from source patients involved in health care worker occupational exposures [Letter]. JAMA 1999;281:1085--6.

156. CDC. Public Health Service task force recommendations for use of antiretroviral drugs in pregnant women infected with HIV-1 for maternal health and for reducing perinatal HIV-1 transmission in the United States. MMWR 1998;47(RR-2).

157. Blanche S, Tardieu M, Rustin P, et al. Persistent mitochondrial dysfunction and perinatal exposure to antiretroviral nucleoside analogues. Lancet 1999;354:1084--9.

158. Smith ME, US Nucleoside Safety Review Working Group. Ongoing nucleoside safety review of HIV exposed children in US studies [Abstract 96]. In: Final program and abstracts for the Second Conference on Global Strategies for the Prevention of HIV Transmission from Mothers to Infants. Montreal, Canada: New York Academy of Sciences, 1999:49.

159. Food and Drug Administration. Important drug warning. Available at <http://www.fda.gov/medwatch/safety/2001/zerit&videx_letter.htm>. Accessed May 9, 2001.

160. Veeder AV, McErlean M, Putnam K, Caldwell WC, Venezia RA. The impact of a rapid HIV test to limit unnecessary post exposure prophylaxis following occupational exposures [Abstract P-S2-66]. In: Program and Abstracts of the 4th Decennial International Conference on Nosocomial and Healthcare-Associated Infections in conjunction with the 10th Annual Meeting of SHEA. Atlanta, GA: CDC, 2000:127.

161. CDC. Guidelines for prevention of transmission of human immunodeficiency virus and hepatitis B virus to health-care and public-safety workers. MMWR 1989;38(No. S-6).

162. Garner JS, Hospital Infection Control Practices Advisory Committee. Guideline for isolation precautions in hospitals. Infect Control Hosp Epidemiol 1996;17:54--80.

163. CDC. Recommendations for preventing transmission of human immunodeficiency virus and hepatitis B virus to patients during exposure-prone invasive procedures. MMWR 1991;40(No. RR-8).

164. Coursaget P, Yvonnet B, Relyveld EH, Barres JL, DiopMar I, Chiron JP. Simultaneous administration of diphtheriatetanuspertussispolio and hepatitis B vaccines in a simplified immunization program: immune response to diphtheria toxoid, tetanus toxoid, pertussis, and hepatitis B surface antigen. Infect Immun 1986;51:784--7.

165. Hadler SC, Francis DP, Maynard JE, et al. Long-term immunogenicity and efficacy of hepatitis B vaccine in homosexual men. N Engl J Med 1986;315:209--14.

166. CDC. Public Health Service inter-agency guidelines for screening donors of blood, plasma, organs, tissues, and semen for evidence of hepatitis B and hepatitis C. MMWR 1991;40(No. RR-4):1--17.

167. Ridzon R, Gallagher K, Ciesielski C, et al. Simultaneous transmission of human immunodeficiency virus and hepatitis C virus from a needle-stick injury. N Engl J Med 1997;336:919--22.

168. Ciesielski CA, Metler RP. Duration of time between exposure and seroconversion in healthcare workers with occupationally acquired infection with human immunodeficiency virus. Am J Med 1997;102(suppl 5B):115--6.

169. Busch MP, Satten GA. Time course of viremia and antibody seroconversion following human immunodeficiency virus exposure. Am J Med 1997;102(suppl 5B):117--24.

170. Rich JD, Merriman NA, Mylonakis E, et al. Misdiagnosis of HIV infection by HIV-1 plasma viral load testing: a case series. Ann Intern Med 1999;130:37--9.

171. Roland ME, Elbeik TA, Martin JN, et al. HIV-1 RNA testing by bDNA and PCR in asymptomatic patients following sexual exposure to HIV [Abstract 776]. In: Program and abstracts of the 7th Conference on Retroviruses and Opportunistic Infections. San Francisco, CA: Foundation for Retrovirology and Human Health in scientific collaboration with the National Institute of Allergy and Infectious Diseases and CDC, 2000:220.

172. Gerberding JL, Henderson DK. Management of occupational exposures to bloodborne pathogens: hepatitis B virus, hepatitis C virus, and human immunodeficiency virus. Clin Inf Dis 1992;14:1179--85.

173. Armstrong K, Gorden R, Santorella G. Occupational exposures of health care workers (HCWs) to human immunodeficiency virus (HIV): stress reactions and counseling interventions. Soc Work Health Care 1995;21:61--80.
174. Henry K, Campbell S, Jackson B, et al. Long-term follow-up of health care workers with work-site exposure to human immunodeficiency virus [Letter]. JAMA 1990;263:1765.
175. AIDS/TB Committee of the Society for Healthcare Epidemiology of America. Management of healthcare workers infected with hepatitis B virus, hepatitis C virus, human immunodeficiency virus, or other bloodborne pathogens. Infect Control Hosp Epidemiol 1997;18:349--63.

TABLE 1. Reported instances of failure of combination drug postexposure prophylaxis to prevent HIV infection in health-care personnel exposed to HIV-infected blood

Report no.	Source of injury	Regimen*	Hours to first dose	Days to onset of retroviral illness	Days to seroconversions[†]	Source patient on antiretrovirals
1[§]	Biopsy needle	ZDV, ddl	0.50	23	23	yes
2[¶]	Hollow needle	ZDV, ddl**	1.50	45	97	no
3[¶]	Large-bore hollow needle	3-drugs[†]	1.50	40	55	yes[§]
4[¶]	Hollow needle	ZDV, 3TC ddl, IDV	0.67	70	83	yes***
5[♯]	Unknown sharp	ddl, d4T NVP[♯]	2.00	42	100	yes***

* ZDV = zidovudine, ddl = didanosine, 3TC = lamivudine, IDV = indinavir, d4T = stavudine, and NVP = nevirapine

[†] By enzyme immunoassay for HIV-1 antibody and Western blot.

[§] Jochimsen EM. Failures of zidovudine postexposure prophylaxis. Am J Med 1997;102(suppl 5B):52–5.

[¶] Lot F, Abiteboul D. Occupational HIV infection in France [Abstract WP-25]. In: Keynote addresses and abstracts of the 4th ICOH International Conference on Occupational Health for Health Care Workers. Montreal, Canada, 1999.

** Report 2: ZDV and ddl taken for 48 hours then changed to ZDV alone.

[†] Report 3: ZDV, 3TC, and IDV taken for 48 hours then changed to d4T, 3TC, and IDV.

[§] HIV isolate tested and determined to be sensitive to antiretroviral agent(s).

[¶] Perdue B, Wolderufael D, Mellors J, Quinn T, Margolick J. HIV-1 transmission by a needlestick injury despite rapid initiation of four-drug postexposure prophylaxis [Abstract 210]. In: Program and abstracts of the 6th Conference on Retroviruses and Opportunistic Infections. Chicago, IL: Foundation for Retrovirology and Human Health in scientific collaboration with the National Institute of Allergy and Infectious Diseases and CDC, 1999:107.

*** HIV isolate tested and determined to be resistant to antiretroviral agent(s).

[♯] Beltrami EM, Luo C-C, Dela Torre N, Cardo DM. HIV transmission after an occupational exposure despite postexposure prophylaxis with a combination drug regimen [Abstract P-S2-62]. In: Program and abstracts of the 4th Decennial International Conference on Nosocomial and Healthcare-Associated Infections in conjunction with the 10th Annual Meeting of SHEA. Atlanta, GA: CDC, 2000:125–6.

[♯] Report 5: ZDV and 3TC taken for one dose then changed to ddl, d4T, and NVP; ddl was discontinued after 3 days because of severe vomiting.

TABLE 2. Primary side effects associated with antiretroviral agents

Antiretroviral class/agent	Primary side effects and toxicities
Nucleoside reverse transcriptase inhibitors (NRTIs)	
Zidovudine (Retrovir™; ZDV; AZT)	anemia, neutropenia, nausea, headache, insomnia, muscle pain, and weakness
Lamivudine (Epivir™; 3TC)	abdominal pain, nausea, diarrhea, rash, and pancreatitis
Stavudine (Zerit™; d4T)	peripheral neuropathy, headache, diarrhea, nausea, insomnia, anorexia, pancreatitis, increased liver function tests (LFTs), anemia, and neutropenia
Didanosine (Videx™; ddI)	pancreatitis, lactic acidosis, neuropathy, diarrhea, abdominal pain, and nausea
Abacavir (Ziagen™; ABC)	nausea, diarrhea, anorexia, abdominal pain, fatigue, headache, insomnia, and hypersensitivity reactions
Nonnucleoside reverse transcriptase inhibitors (NNRTIs)	
Nevirapine (Viramune™; NVP)	rash (including cases of Stevens-Johnson syndrome), fever, nausea, headache, hepatitis, and increased LFTs
Delavirdine (Rescriptor™; DLV)	rash (including cases of Stevens-Johnson syndrome), nausea, diarrhea, headache, fatigue, and increased LFTs
Efavirenz (Sustiva™; EFV)	rash (including cases of Stevens-Johnson syndrome), insomnia, somnolence, dizziness, trouble concentrating, and abnormal dreaming
Protease inhibitors (PIs)	
Indinavir (Crixivan™; IDV)	nausea, abdominal pain, nephrolithiasis, and indirect hyperbilirubinemia
Nelfinavir (Viracept™; NFV)	diarrhea, nausea, abdominal pain, weakness, and rash
Ritonavir (Norvir™; RTV)	weakness, diarrhea, nausea, circumoral paresthesia, taste alteration, and increased cholesterol and triglycerides
Saquinavir (Fortovase™; SQV)	diarrhea, abdominal pain, nausea, hyperglycemia, and increased LFTs
Amprenavir (Agenerase™; AMP)	nausea, diarrhea, rash, circumoral paresthesia, taste alteration, and depression
Lopinavir/Ritonavir (Kaletra™)	diarrhea, fatigue, headache, nausea, and increased cholesterol and triglycerides

BOX 1. Recommendations for the contents of the occupational exposure report

- date and time of exposure;
- details of the procedure being performed, including where and how the exposure occurred; if related to a sharp device, the type and brand of device and how and when in the course of handling the device the exposure occurred;
- details of the exposure, including the type and amount of fluid or material and the severity of the exposure (e.g., for a percutaneous exposure, depth of injury and whether fluid was injected; for a skin or mucous membrane exposure, the estimated volume of material and the condition of the skin [e.g., chapped, abraded, intact]);
- details about the exposure source (e.g., whether the source material contained HBV, HCV, or HIV; if the source is HIV-infected, the stage of disease, history of antiretroviral therapy, viral load, and antiretroviral resistance information, if known);
- details about the exposed person (e.g., hepatitis B vaccination and vaccine-response status); and
- details about counseling, postexposure management, and follow-up.

BOX 2. Factors to consider in assessing the need for follow-up of occupational exposures

- **Type of exposure**
  - Percutaneous injury
  - Mucous membrane exposure
  - Nonintact skin exposure
  - Bites resulting in blood exposure to either person involved

- **Type and amount of fluid/tissue**
  - Blood
  - Fluids containing blood
  - Potentially infectious fluid or tissue (semen; vaginal secretions; and cerebrospinal, synovial, pleural, peritoneal, pericardial, and amniotic fluids)
  - Direct contact with concentrated virus

- **Infectious status of source**
  - Presence of HBsAg
  - Presence of HCV antibody
  - Presence of HIV antibody

- **Susceptibility of exposed person**
  - Hepatitis B vaccine and vaccine response status
  - HBV, HCV, and HIV immune status

BOX 3. Evaluation of occupational exposure sources

Known sources
- Test known sources for HBsAg, anti-HCV, and HIV antibody
  - Direct virus assays for routine screening of source patients are **not** recommended
  - Consider using a rapid HIV-antibody test
  - If the source person is **not** infected with a bloodborne pathogen, baseline testing or further follow-up of the exposed person is **not** necessary
- For sources whose infection status remains unknown (e.g., the source person refuses testing), consider medical diagnoses, clinical symptoms, and history of risk behaviors
- Do not test discarded needles for bloodborne pathogens

Unknown sources
- For unknown sources, evaluate the likelihood of exposure to a source at high risk for infection
  - Consider likelihood of bloodborne pathogen infection among patients in the exposure setting

TABLE 3. Recommended postexposure prophylaxis for exposure to hepatitis B virus

Vaccination and antibody response status of exposed workers*	Treatment		
	Source HBsAg[¹] positive	Source HBsAg[¹] negative	Source unknown or not available for testing
Unvaccinated	HBIG[§] x 1 and initiate HB vaccine series[¶]	Initiate HB vaccine series	Initiate HB vaccine series
Previously vaccinated			
Known responder**	No treatment	No treatment	No treatment
Known nonresponder[††]	HBIG x 1 and initiate revaccination or HBIG x 2[§]	No treatment	If known high risk source, treat as if source were HBsAg positive
Antibody response unknown	Test exposed person for anti-HBs[¶] 1. If adequate,** no treatment is necessary 2. If inadequate,[††] administer HBIG x 1 and vaccine booster	No treatment	Test exposed person for anti-HBs 1. If adequate,[¶] no treatment is necessary 2. If inadequate,[¶] administer vaccine booster and recheck titer in 1–2 months

* Persons who have previously been infected with HBV are immune to reinfection and do not require postexposure prophylaxis.

[¹] Hepatitis B surface antigen.

[§] Hepatitis B immune globulin; dose is 0.06 mL/kg intramuscularly.

[¶] Hepatitis B vaccine.

** A responder is a person with adequate levels of serum antibody to HBsAg (i.e., anti-HBs ≥ 10 mIU/mL).

[†] A nonresponder is a person with inadequate response to vaccination (i.e., serum anti-HBs < 10 mIU/mL).

[§] The option of giving one dose of HBIG and reinitiating the vaccine series is preferred for nonresponders who have not completed a second 3-dose vaccine series. For persons who previously completed a second vaccine series but failed to respond, two doses of HBIG are preferred.

[¶] Antibody to HBsAg.

TABLE 5. Recommended HIV postexposure prophylaxis for mucous membrane exposures and nonintact skin* exposures

Exposure type	Infection status of source				
	HIV-Positive Class 1†	HIV-Positive Class 2†	Source of unknown HIV status§	Unknown source¶	HIV-Negative
Small volume**	Consider basic 2-drug PEP††	Recommend basic 2-drug PEP	Generally, no PEP warranted; however, consider basic 2-drug PEP†† for source with HIV risk factors§§	Generally, no PEP warranted; however, consider basic 2-drug PEP†† in settings where exposure to HIV-infected persons is likely	No PEP warranted
Large volume¶¶	Recommend basic 2-drug PEP	Recommend expanded 3-drug PEP	Generally, no PEP warranted; however, consider basic 2-drug PEP†† for source with HIV risk factors§§	Generally, no PEP warranted; however, consider basic 2-drug PEP†† in settings where exposure to HIV-infected persons is likely	No PEP warranted

* For skin exposures, follow-up is indicated only if there is evidence of compromised skin integrity (e.g., dermatitis, abrasion, or open wound).

† HIV-Positive, Class 1 — asymptomatic HIV infection or known low viral load (e.g., <1,500 RNA copies/mL). HIV-Positive, Class 2 — symptomatic HIV infection, AIDS, acute seroconversion, or known high viral load. If drug resistance is a concern, obtain expert consultation. Initiation of postexposure prophylaxis (PEP) should not be delayed pending expert consultation, and, because expert consultation alone cannot substitute for face-to-face counseling, resources should be available to provide immediate evaluation and follow-up care for all exposures.

§ Source of unknown HIV status (e.g., deceased source person with no samples available for HIV testing).

¶ Unknown source (e.g., splash from inappropriately disposed blood).

** Small volume (i.e., a few drops).

†† The designation, "consider PEP," indicates that PEP is optional and should be based on an individualized decision between the exposed person and the treating clinician.

§ If PEP is offered and taken and the source is later determined to be HIV-negative, PEP should be discontinued.

¶ Large volume (i.e., major blood splash).

BOX 4. Situations for which expert* consultation for HIV postexposure prophylaxis is advised

- Delayed (i.e., later than 24–36 hours) exposure report
  - the interval after which there is no benefit from postexposure prophylaxis (PEP) is undefined

- Unknown source (e.g., needle in sharps disposal container or laundry)
  - decide use of PEP on a case-by-case basis
  - consider the severity of the exposure and the epidemiologic likelihood of HIV exposure
  - do not test needles or other sharp instruments for HIV

- Known or suspected pregnancy in the exposed person
  - does not preclude the use of optimal PEP regimens
  - do not deny PEP solely on the basis of pregnancy

- Resistance of the source virus to antiretroviral agents
  - influence of drug resistance on transmission risk is unknown
  - selection of drugs to which the source person's virus is unlikely to be resistant is recommended, if the source person's virus is known or suspected to be resistant to ≥ 1 of the drugs considered for the PEP regimen
  - resistance testing of the source person's virus at the time of the exposure is not recommended

- Toxicity of the initial PEP regimen
  - adverse symptoms, such as nausea and diarrhea are common with PEP
  - symptoms often can be managed without changing the PEP regimen by prescribing antimotility and/or antiemetic agents
  - modification of dose intervals (i.e., administering a lower dose of drug more frequently throughout the day, as recommended by the manufacturer), in other situations, might help alleviate symptoms

*Local experts and/or the National Clinicians' Post-Exposure Prophylaxis Hotline (PEPline [1-888-448-4911]).

BOX 5. Occupational exposure management resources

National Clinicians' Postexposure Prophylaxis Hotline (PEPline) Run by University of California–San Francisco/San Francisco General Hospital staff; supported by the Health Resources and Services Administration Ryan White CARE Act, HIV/AIDS Bureau, AIDS Education and Training Centers, and CDC.	Phone: (888) 448-4911 Internet: <http://www.ucsf.edu/hivcntr>
Needlestick! A website to help clinicians manage and document occupational blood and body fluid exposures. Developed and maintained by the University of California, Los Angeles (UCLA), Emergency Medicine Center, UCLA School of Medicine, and funded in party by CDC and the Agency for Healthcare Research and Quality.	Internet: <http://www.needlestick.mednet.ucla.edu>
Hepatitis Hotline.	Phone: (888) 443-7232 Internet: <http://www.cdc.gov/hepatitis>
Reporting to CDC: Occupationally acquired HIV infections and failures of PEP.	Phone: (800) 893-0485
HIV Antiretroviral Pregnancy Registry.	Phone: (800) 258-4263 Fax: (800) 800-1052 Address: 1410 Commonwealth Drive Suite 215 Wilmington, NC 28405 Internet: <http://www.glaxowellcome.com/preg_reg/antiretroviral>

BOX 5. (*Continued*) Occupational exposure management resources

Food and Drug Administration
Report unusual or severe toxicity
to antiretroviral agents.
	Phone: (800) 332-1088
	Address:
	  MedWatch
	  HF-2, FDA
	  5600 Fishers Lane
	  Rockville, MD 20857
	Internet:
	     <http://www.fda.gov/medwatch>

HIV/AIDS Treatment Information Service.	Internet: <http://www.hivatis.org>

Disclaimer All *MMWR* HTML versions of articles are electronic conversions from ASCII text into HTML. This conversion may have resulted in character translation or format errors in the HTML version. Users should not rely on this HTML document, but are referred to the electronic PDF version and/or the original *MMWR* paper copy for the official text, figures, and tables. An original paper copy of this issue can be obtained from the Superintendent of Documents, U.S. Government Printing Office (GPO), Washington, DC 20402-9371; telephone: (202) 512-1800. Contact GPO for current prices.

APPENDIX C

SOURCES OF ADDITIONAL INFORMATION

FEDERAL

AGENCY	NOTES
United States Fire Administration National Fire Programs 16825 South Seton Avenue Emmitsburg, MD 21727 http://www.usfa.fema.gov/	Developed *Guide to Managing an Emergency Service Infection Control Program* Two-day course: *Infection Control for Emergency Response Personnel: The Supervisor's Role*
U.S. Department of Health and Human Services Public Health Service, Centers for Disease Control 1600 Clifton Rd. Atlanta, GA 30333 http://www.cdc.gov	Conducts ongoing research Oversees National Prevention Information Network Publishes MMWR
Morbidity and Mortality Weekly Report Epidemiology Program Office MS C-08 Centers for Disease Control and Prevention 1600 Clifton Rd. Atlanta, GA 30333 http://www2.cdc.gov/mmwr/	Weekly reports from CDC on communicable diseases
National Highway Traffic Safety Administration Division of EMS Department of Transportation 400 7th Street, N.W. Washington, D.C. 20590 http://www.nhtsa.dot.gov/people/injury/ems/	Developed *A Leadership Guide to Quality Improvement for Emergency Medical Services Systems*
U.S. Department of Labor Occupational Health & Safety Administration Office of Public Affairs, Room N3647 200 Constitution Avenue, N.W. Washington, D.C. 20210 http://www.osha.gov/	29 CFR Part 1910.1030 *Occupational Exposure to Bloodborne Pathogens; Final Rule* (http://www.osha-slc.gov/Preamble/Blood_data/BLOOD9.html)

STATE

Public Health Agencies	Liaison with CDC Enforce CDC guidelines
Fire and EMS Agencies	Liaison with USFA and NFA Sponsor training on infection control

AGENCY	NOTES
State OSHA (where applicable)	Enforce OSHA regulations and CDC guidelines http://www.osha-slc.gov/fso/osp/ provides links to State OSHA contacts

LOCAL

AGENCY	NOTES
Public Health Agencies	Liaison with State, public, health agencies Screening, testing, evaluation, immunization, and treatment capabilities
Regional EMS Agencies	Liaison to State EMS agencies
Hospitals	Access to current information on infection control Notify responders of possible exposures

OTHER HELPFUL WEB SITES

http://www.osha-slc.gov/FedReg_osha_pdf/FED20010118A.pdf	29 CFR Part 1910, *Occupational Exposure to Bloodborne Pathogens; Needlesticks and Other Sharps Injuries; Final Rule*
http://www.osha-slc.gov/SLTC/needlestick/saferneedledevices/saferneedledevices.html	*Safer Needle Devices: Protecting Health Care Workers* (OSHA)
http://www.osha-slc.gov/html/hotfoias/tib/TIB19990412.html	*Technical Information Bulletin - Potential for Allergy to Natural Rubber Latex Gloves and other Natural Rubber Products* (OSHA)
http://www.osha-slc.gov/OshDoc/Directive_data/CPL_2-2_44D.html	CPL 2-2.44D - *Enforcement Procedures for the Occupational Exposure to Bloodborne Pathogens* (OSHA)

AGENCY	NOTES
http://www.cdc.gov/ncidod/diseases/hepatitis/index.htm	*Viral Hepatitis* (CDC)
http://www.cdc.gov/hiv/pubs/facts/hivtb.pdf	*The Deadly Intersection between TB and HIV* (CDC)
http://www.cdc.gov/epo/mmwr/preview/mmwrhtml/00035909.htm	*Guidelines for Preventing the Transmission of Mycobacterium tuberculosis in Health-Care Facilities, 1994* (CDC)
http://www.cdc.gov/epo/mmwr/preview/mmwrhtml/00053391.htm	*Measles, Mumps, and Rubella -- Vaccine Use and Strategies for Elimination of Measles, Rubella, and Congenital Rubella Syndrome and Control of Mumps: Recommendations of the Advisory Committee on Immunization Practices (ACIP)* (CDC)
http://www.cdc.gov/epo/mmwr/preview/mmwrhtml/top	*Prevention and Control of Meningococcal Disease* (CDC)
http://www.osha-slc.gov/OshStd_data/1910_0134.html	29 CFR *Respiratory Protection* (OSHA 1910.134)
http://www.osha-slc.gov/OshDoc/Directive_data/CPL_2-2_44D.html	*Enforcement Procedures for the Occupational Exposure to Bloodborne Pathogens* (OSHA Directive CPL2-2.44D)
http://www.osha.gov/oshpubs/osha3130.pdf	*Occupational Exposure to Bloodborne Pathogens – Precautions for Emergency Responders* ((OSHA 3130 Revised)

NATIONAL ORGANIZATIONS

Association for Professionals in Infection Control
1275 K. St. N.W., Suite 1000
Washington, D.C. 20005-4006
(202) 789-1890
http://www.apic.org/

Published *APIC Text of Infection Control and Epidemiology*

AGENCY	NOTES
National Fire Protection Association Batterymarch Park Quincy, MA 02269-9904 (800) 344-3555 (to order documents) http://www.nfpa.org	NFPA 1581, *Standard on Fire Department Infection Control Program*
International Association of Firefighters Department of Occupational Health & Safety 1750 New York Avenue, N.W. Washington, D.C. 20006 (202) 737-8484 http://www.iaff.org/iaff/Health_Safety/health_safety.html	Develops knowledge within the fire service so firefighters, paramedics and EMT's can recognize and control the safety and health hazards associated with the profession
International Association of Fire Chiefs 1329 18th St., N.W. Washington, D.C. 20036 (202) 833-3420 http://www.iafc.org/	Promotes infection control policies and practices
National Prevention Information Network P.O. Box 6003 Rockville, MD 20850 800-458-5231 http://www.cdc.gov/hiv/hivinfo/npin.htm	Formerly AIDS Information Clearinghouse. Distributes HIV/AIDS, STD, and TB information